# RHYTHM AND BEATS

## THE COMPLETE EKG INTERPRETATION RESOURCE

ROCK LOUIS

# TABLE OF CONTENTS

# PREFACE

Dear Reader,

The heartbeat is the drumbeat of life – a complex symphony of electrical impulses that sustain us from our first breath to our last. The electrocardiogram (EKG) stands as one of the greatest inventions in the history of medicine, a simple yet profound tool that allows us a glimpse into the heart's function and its many rhythms.

In the journey of creating "The Heart's Rhythms:" **Rhythm and Beats: The Complete EKG Interpretation Resource,"** I aimed to distill the complexity of cardiac electrophysiology into a format that is accessible and engaging. This book is born out of my experiences as an educator and clinician, where I have seen the need for a clear, comprehensive, and approachable guide on this subject.

Whether you are a student stepping into the world of healthcare, a practicing Cardiograph Technician (Monitor Technician), a nurse, a paramedic seeking to refresh your skills or even a curious individual fascinated by the wonders of human physiology, this book is for you. My hope is that it will not only serve as an educational resource but also inspire you to appreciate the marvels of the human heart.

Within these pages lies a journey through the landscape of cardiac rhythms – from the normal to the life-threatening. It is a path that will challenge you, but I assure you it is a rewarding one. The knowledge you gain here has the power to make a difference in patients' lives, perhaps even to save them.

So, as you turn these pages and embark on this learning adventure, remember that each chapter builds on the last, each concept a stepping stone to the next. I encourage you to engage with the material actively, ask questions, and seek to understand not just the 'how' but also the 'why' behind each rhythm.

Thank you for choosing this guide as your companion on the path to mastering EKG interpretation. May the knowledge you gain empower you and the lives you touch.

With heartfelt beats,

Rock Louis
Certified Cardiograph Technician
Master's in accounting and financial management

# I-INTRODUCTION TO ELECTROCARDIOGRAM (EKG/ECG)

1. Definition and Basic Principles
2. Historical Overview and Invention

## 1-Definition

An Electrocardiogram (EKG or ECG) is a medical test that records the electrical activity of the heart. This non-invasive procedure is essential in diagnosing and monitoring heart conditions, measuring heart rate, and detecting any irregularities in heart rhythm and structure.

## 2-Historical Perspective and Invention

The development of the EKG has been a cornerstone in cardiology. Pioneered by Willem Einthoven in the early 20th century, the EKG evolved from a simple string galvanometer to the sophisticated systems used today. Einthoven's work not only led to the creation of the standard EKG but also laid the groundwork for future cardiac research and diagnosis.

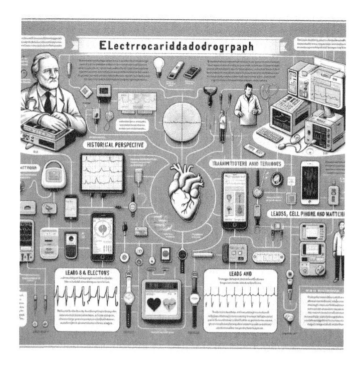

# II-EKG DEVICES AND TECHNOLOGY

1. Standard EKG Machines
2. Portable and Wearable Devices: Transmitters, Cell Phones, and Watches

## 1-Standard EKG Machines

EKG technology has diversified over the years. Today, it ranges from sophisticated hospital-based machines, which provide comprehensive cardiac monitoring, to compact, portable devices used in clinics and home settings. These devices vary in the number of leads, portability, and functionality, catering to different diagnostic needs.

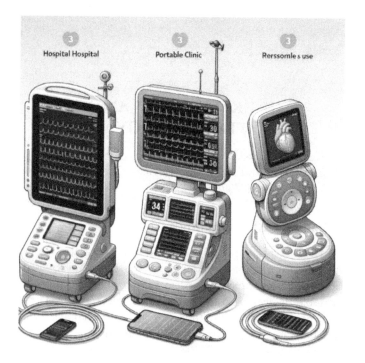

1. **Hospital-Based EKG Machine:** This image shows the 'Advanced Hospital EKG System,' a large and sophisticated EKG machine with multiple leads, high-resolution displays, and advanced diagnostic features, typically found in hospital settings.

2. **Portable Clinic EKG Device**: The second image depicts a 'Compact Clinic EKG Device,' which is smaller and portable, designed for clinical use. It demonstrates the device's compact size yet compatibility with multiple leads, ideal for outpatient clinics and primary care settings.

3. Home-Use EKG Device: The third image illustrates a 'Personal EKG Monitor,' very compact and user-friendly, intended for personal home use. It highlights the device's simple interface and portability, suitable for patients who need regular cardiac activity tracking at home.

## 2-Portable and Wearable Devices: Transmitters, Cell Phones, Watches

The advent of mobile technology has revolutionized EKG monitoring. Smartwatches and cell phones equipped with EKG transmitters now allow for continuous, real-time heart monitoring. These devices are particularly useful for detecting intermittent cardiac arrhythmias and for remote patient monitoring.

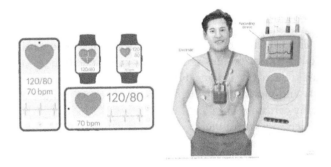

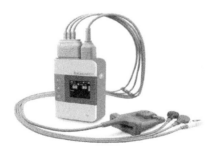

# III-FUNDAMENTALS EKG LEADS AND ELECTRODES

1. Leads and Electrodes Overview
2. Lead Systems in EKG
3. Placement

## 1. Leads and Electrodes Overview

The Electrocardiogram (EKG) is a vital tool in cardiac diagnostics, providing a graphical representation of the heart's electrical activity. Fundamental to this process are leads and electrodes, which work together to capture and display cardiac rhythms.

Electrodes are adhesive patches attached to the skin that detect electrical signals from the heart. Leads, on the other hand, refer to the electrical pathways between these electrodes, through which the heart's activity is transmitted and interpreted by the EKG machine

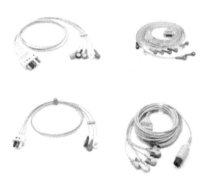

## 2-Lead Systems in EKG

Electrocardiography (EKG or ECG) utilizes various lead systems to provide views of the electrical activity of the heart from different angles. These systems include limb leads, augmented leads, and precordial (chest) leads, each offering unique insights into cardiac function.

Limb Leads

- Standard Bipolar Limb Leads (I, II, III):
    - Lead I: Measures the electrical potential between the right arm (RA) and left arm (LA). It views the lateral wall of the left ventricle.
    - Lead II: Measures between the right arm and left leg (LL). It's often the best lead for rhythm analysis as it views the heart's electrical axis.
    - Lead III: Measures between the left arm and left leg. It provides a view of the inferior portion of the heart.
- Configuration: These leads form Einthoven's triangle, a conceptual representation of the heart's electrical activity in the frontal plane.

Augmented Limb Leads (aVR, aVL, aVF)

- Augmented Unipolar Limb Leads:
    - aVR (Right Arm): Views the heart from the right shoulder.
    - aVL (Left Arm): Offers a view of the lateral wall of the left ventricle.
    - aVF (Left Foot): Provides a perspective of the heart's inferior wall.
- Purpose: These leads augment the electrical signals from the limbs to create a more comprehensive view of the heart's electrical activity in the frontal plane.

Precordial (Chest) Leads

- Leads V1 to V6:

- Placed in specific locations on the chest wall.
- V1 and V2: Positioned on either side of the sternum in the fourth intercostal space, providing views of the septal area of the heart.
- V3 and V4: V3 between V2 and V4, and V4 at the mid-clavicular line in the fifth intercostal space, focusing on the anterior wall of the left ventricle.
- V5 and V6: V5 at the anterior axillary line and V6 at the mid-axillary line, both in line with V4, giving lateral views of the left ventricle.

- Purpose: Precordial leads are crucial for detecting conditions affecting the anterior, septal, and lateral walls of the left ventricle, such as myocardial infarction.

12-Lead EKG

- Combination: The standard 12-lead EKG combines all these leads (3 limb leads, 3 augmented limb leads, and 6 precordial leads) to give a comprehensive view of the heart's electrical activity.
- Applications: Widely used for diagnosing arrhythmias, myocardial infarction, and other cardiac abnormalities.

Summary

The lead systems in an EKG provide multiple perspectives of the heart's electrical activity, enabling detailed analysis and diagnosis of cardiac conditions. The combination of limb and precordial leads in a 12-lead EKG offers a complete picture, crucial for accurate cardiac assessment and treatment planning.

# 3-Placement

## 3-Lead and 5-Lead EKG Placement

Understanding the placement of leads in a 3-lead and 5-lead EKG setup is crucial for accurate cardiac monitoring and interpretation. These setups are commonly used in different clinical settings, including ambulatory monitoring and bedside telemetry.

## 3-Lead EKG Placement

Purpose: Used for basic heart rate and rhythm monitoring. Common in pre-hospital settings, during transportation, and in emergency situations.

Leads: Consists of three electrodes – typically labeled as RA (right arm), LA (left arm), and LL (left leg).

Placement:

- RA (Red): Placed on the right arm, below the clavicle and near the shoulder.
- LA (Yellow): Placed on the left arm, below the clavicle, and near the shoulder.
- LL (Green): Placed on the left leg, below the costal margin on the torso or on the upper thigh.
- Note: The right leg (RL) lead serves as a ground and is not used for monitoring but can be placed on the right leg or abdomen for stabilization of baseline.

Lead Configurations: The three leads provide different views of the heart (Lead I, Lead II, and Lead III).

## 5-Lead EKG Placement

Purpose: Provides more comprehensive heart monitoring than a 3-lead EKG. Common in hospital settings for continuous monitoring of patients.

Leads: In addition to the three leads used in the 3-lead setup, two additional leads (V1 and V2 or V5) are added.

Placement:

- RA (Red), LA (Yellow), and LL (Green): Same as in the 3-lead setup.

- V1 Lead (Brown): Placed in the fourth intercostal space to the right of the sternum.
- V2 or V5 Lead (Black or White): V2 is placed in the fourth intercostal space to the left of the sternum. Alternatively, V5 can be placed in the fifth intercostal space at the mid-clavicular line on the left side of the chest.

Lead Configurations: In addition to Leads I, II, and III, the 5-lead setup provides additional precordial views (V1 and either V2 or V5), offering more information about the heart's electrical activity, particularly the anterior and lateral walls.

### Key Points

Choice of Setup: The choice between a 3-lead and a 5-lead setup depends on the clinical situation and the level of monitoring required.

Accuracy: Correct placement of leads is crucial for accurate EKG interpretation and the detection of arrhythmias or ischemic changes.

Clinical Application: While 3-lead EKGs are sufficient for basic monitoring, 5-lead EKGs provide a more detailed view of the heart's electrical activity and are preferred in settings where more comprehensive monitoring is necessary.

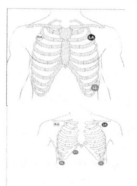

Both 3-lead and 5-lead EKG setups are essential tools in cardiac monitoring, each serving specific roles in different clinical contexts.

## Placement of 12 EKG Leads

Proper placement of EKG leads is crucial for accurate interpretation:

## Standard Limb Leads (I, II, III)

- Lead I: Between the right and left arm.
- Lead II: From the right arm to the left leg.
- Lead III: From the left arm to the left leg.

## Augmented Limb Leads (aVR, aVL, aVF)

- aVR: On the right arm.
- aVL: On the left arm.
- aVF: On the left leg.

## Precordial (Chest) Leads (V1-V6)

- V1: 4th intercostal space, right of the sternum.
- V2: 4th intercostal space, left of the sternum.
- V3: Between V2 and V4.
- V4: 5th intercostal space, mid-clavicular line.
- V5: Level with V4, anterior axillary line.
- V6: Level with V5, mid-axillary line.

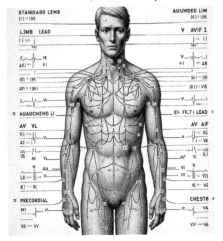

# IV-HEART OVERVIEW

1. Anatomy and Physiology
2. The Electrical Conduction System of the Heart

## 1. Anatomy and Physiology

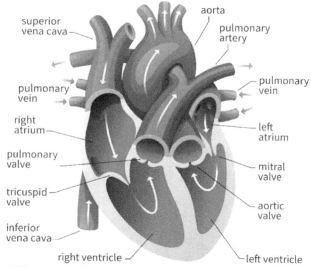

The human heart, a vital organ in the circulatory system, functions primarily as a pump to circulate blood throughout the body. Here's a brief overview of its anatomy and physiology:

Structure

- Four Chambers: Comprises two atria (upper chambers) and two ventricles (lower chambers).
    - Atria: Receive blood returning to the heart. The right atrium receives deoxygenated

blood from the body, while the left atrium receives oxygenated blood from the lungs.

- Ventricles: Pump blood out of the heart. The right ventricle pumps blood to the lungs for oxygenation, and the left ventricle pumps oxygenated blood to the body.
- Valves: Four valves regulate blood flow through the heart.
- Tricuspid Valve: Between the right atrium and right ventricle.
- Pulmonary Valve: Between the right ventricle and pulmonary artery.
- Mitral Valve: Between the left atrium and left ventricle.
- Aortic Valve: Between the left ventricle and the aorta.
- Major Blood Vessels:
  - Aorta: Carries oxygenated blood from the left ventricle to the body.
  - Pulmonary Arteries: Transport deoxygenated blood from the right ventricle to the lungs.
  - Superior and Inferior Vena Cava: Bring deoxygenated blood from the body back to the right atrium.

Function
- Blood Circulation: The heart circulates blood through two pathways: the systemic circuit (body) and the pulmonary circuit (lungs).
- Oxygen Exchange: Blood is oxygenated in the lungs and then distributed to the body's tissues, providing essential oxygen and nutrients.
- Cardiac Cycle: Involves the coordinated contraction (systole) and relaxation (diastole) of the heart's chambers.

## 2-Electrical Conduction System of the Heart

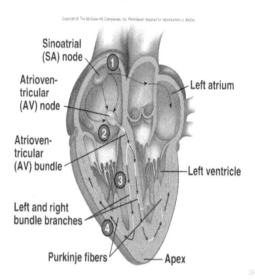

# Conducting System of Heart

The heart's electrical conduction system is a complex network that ensures coordinated heartbeats. This system includes:

**Sinoatrial (SA) Node**: Located in the right atrium's upper wall, the SA node generates electrical impulses, setting the pace for the heart rate. It's often referred to as the heart's natural pacemaker. The SA node typically generates impulses at a rate of about 60 to 100 beats per minute in a healthy adult at rest.

**Atrioventricular (AV) Node**: Positioned at the lower end of the right atrium, near the atrial septum. This node acts as a gatekeeper, slightly delaying the electrical impulse from the SA node, allowing the ventricles to fill with blood before they contract. If the SA node fails, the

AV node can act as a pacemaker with a slower rate called escape rate, usually around 40 to 60 beats per minute.

**Bundle of His**: After passing through the AV node, the impulse travels along the Bundle of His, a collection of heart muscle cells specialized for electrical conduction. This bundle is located in the interventricular septum. In case both the SA and AV nodes fail, the Bundle of His and bundle branches can initiate impulses at an even slower escape rate, typically 20 to 40 beats per minute.

**Right and Left Bundle Branches:** The Bundle of His divides into these branches. The right branch sends impulses to the right ventricle, and the left branch sends impulses to the left ventricle.

**Purkinje Fibers**: Extending from the bundle branches, these fibers spread throughout the ventricular walls. They rapidly conduct the electrical impulse, triggering a coordinated contraction of the ventricles. If all higher centers fail, the Purkinje fibers can generate an escape heart rate of 15 to 40 beats per minute.

# V-BASICS OF HEART RATE AND RHYTHMS

1. Understanding Heartbeat
2. Heart Rate

## 1-Understanding the Heartbeat

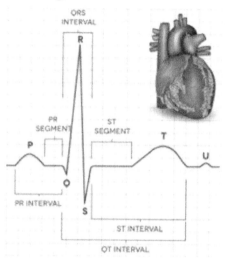

A heartbeat is a complex process that involves the coordinated contraction and relaxation of the heart muscle, allowing it to pump blood throughout the body. It is initiated and regulated by the heart's electrical conduction system. Here's a detailed explanation of how a heartbeat occurs:

### Initiation at the Sinoatrial (SA) Node:

The heartbeat begins at the SA node, located in the right atrium. This node generates an electrical impulse, acting as the heart's natural pacemaker.

The SA node sets the pace of the heart, typically between 60 to 100 beats per minute in a resting adult.

### Atrial Contraction:

The electrical impulse from the SA node causes the atria (the upper chambers of the heart) to contract.

This contraction pushes blood into the ventricles (the lower chambers of the heart).

On an ECG, this atrial contraction is represented by the **P wave**.

### Impulse Delay at the Atrioventricular (AV) Node:

The impulse travels from the SA node to the AV node, located between the atria and ventricles.

The AV node briefly delays the impulse, allowing the ventricles to fully fill with blood from the atria.

### Ventricular Contraction:

From the AV node, the impulse travels down the Bundle of His and through the right and left bundle branches to the Purkinje fibers.

This network rapidly spreads the impulse throughout the ventricles, causing them to contract.

This contraction pumps blood out of the heart – to the lungs from the right ventricle and to the rest of the body from the left ventricle.

The ventricular contraction is seen on the ECG as the QRS complex.

### Ventricular Relaxation:

After contracting, the ventricles relax and repolarize (reset electrically) to prepare for the next heartbeat.

This relaxation and repolarization are represented by the **T wave** on the ECG.

### Heartbeat Cycle:

The entire process from the initiation of the impulse at the SA node to the relaxation of the ventricles constitutes one heartbeat.

The cycle then repeats, continuously pumping blood throughout the body.

## Depolarization and Repolarization

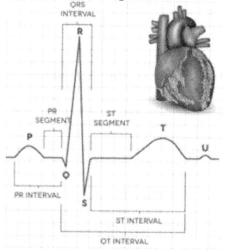

### Depolarization:

**Definition**: Depolarization is the process by which heart muscle cells change electrically. It occurs when positively charged ions, mainly sodium (Na+), rapidly move into a heart cell, causing the inside of the cell to become more positively charged compared to the outside.

**Role in Heartbeat**: In the heart, depolarization triggers the contraction of heart muscle cells. It begins in the sinoatrial (SA) node, spreads through the atria (causing atrial contraction), passes to the atrioventricular (AV) node, then travels down the Bundle of His, through the bundle branches, and along the Purkinje fibers, leading to the contraction of the ventricles.

**ECG Correlation**: On an ECG, atrial depolarization is represented by the P wave, and ventricular depolarization is represented by the **QRS complex.**

### Repolarization:

**Definition:** Repolarization is the process of returning the heart cell to its resting state. It involves the movement of potassium ions (K+) out of the cell, making the inside of the cell more negatively charged compared to the outside.

**Role in Heartbeat**: Repolarization allows the heart muscle cells to relax and prepare for the next cycle of depolarization and contraction. In the ventricles, repolarization must occur before they can contract again.

**ECG Correlation**: In an ECG, ventricular repolarization is represented by the **T wave.** Atrial repolarization also occurs but is usually masked by the larger QRS complex.

## 2-Heart Rate

Heart rate refers to the number of times the heart beats per minute (bpm). It's a crucial measure of heart health and function. Various methods can be used to calculate heart rate, especially during EKG interpretation:

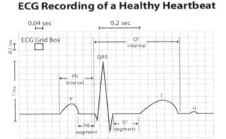

**ECG Recording of a Healthy Heartbeat**

## Rate Calculation:

Method: Count the number of QRS complexes in a 6-second strip and multiply by 10 to estimate beats per minute (bpm). Alternatively, measure the distance between R waves in small squares (each representing 0.04 seconds) and apply the 1500 method (1500 divided by the number of small squares between R waves). Or use EKG Rate Determination Chart.

EKG RATE DETERMINATION CHART

| Spaces | Rate | Spaces | Rate | Spaces | Rate | Spaces | Rate |
|---|---|---|---|---|---|---|---|
| 3 | 500 | 12.5 | 120 | 22 | 68 | 32 | 47 |
| 3.5 | 428 | 13 | 115 | 23 | 65 | 32.5 | 46 |
| 4 | 374 | 13.5 | 111 | 23.5 | 63 | 33 | 45 |
| 4.5 | 334 | 14 | 107 | 24 | 62 | 34 | 44 |
| 5 | 300 | 15 | 100 | 24.5 | 61 | 35 | 43 |
| 5.5 | 273 | 15.5 | 97 | 25 | 60 | 36 | 42 |
| 6 | 250 | 16 | 94 | 25.5 | 59 | 37 | 41 |
| 7 | 214 | 16.5 | 91 | 26 | 58 | 37.5 | 40 |
| 7.5 | 200 | 17 | 88 | 26.5 | 57 | 38 | 39 |
| 8 | 188 | 17.5 | 86 | 27 | 56 | 39 | 38 |
| 8.5 | 176 | 18 | 83 | 27.5 | 55 | 40 | 37 |
| 9 | 167 | 18.5 | 81 | 28 | 54 | 42 | 36 |
| 9.5 | 158 | 19 | 79 | 28.5 | 53 | 43 | 35 |
| 10 | 150 | 19.5 | 77 | 29 | 52 | 44 | 34 |
| 10.5 | 143 | 20 | 75 | 29.5 | 51 | 46 | 33 |
| 11 | 136 | 20.5 | 73 | 30 | 50 | 47 | 32 |
| 11.5 | 130 | 21 | 71 | 30.5 | 49 | 48 | 31 |
| 12 | 125 | 21.5 | 70 | 31 | 48 | 50 | 30 |

Using an EKG rate determination chart, often referred to as an EKG ruler or rate chart, is a convenient way to calculate heart rate from an EKG strip. Here's how to use this tool:

Steps to Use an EKG Rate Determination Chart

Align the Chart with the EKG Strip:

Start by aligning one of the vertical lines on the rate chart with a prominent R wave on the EKG strip.

Count the R Waves:

The chart typically has a sequence of numbers or marks that represent heart rates at regular intervals. After aligning the first line with an R wave, look to see where the next R wave falls on the chart.

### Read the Heart Rate:

The number or mark on the chart where the next R wave aligns will indicate the heart rate. For instance, if the next R wave aligns with the number 75 on the chart, the heart rate is 75 beats per minute.

Regular vs. Irregular Rhythms:

For regular rhythms, this method works well as the R waves should consistently align with the numbers or marks on the chart.

For irregular rhythms, the rate determination chart may not be as accurate because the R-R intervals (the distance between consecutive R waves) vary. In such cases, averaging the rate over a longer strip or using other methods like the 1500 method or 6-second rule might be more appropriate.

Considerations:

Ensure the EKG strip speed is standard (usually 25 mm (about 0.98 in)/sec) as the rate chart is calibrated for this speed.

Some rate charts also include scales for calculating PR intervals, QRS duration, and QT intervals.

Practical Tips

Familiarity with the Chart: Different rate charts might have slightly different designs or scales, so it's important to be familiar with the specific chart you are using.

Accuracy: While rate charts are convenient, they might not be as accurate as manual calculations, especially for complex rhythms. They are best used for quick estimations.

**Manual Counting**:

Method: Feel the pulse at a point like the wrist or neck, count the number of beats for 15 seconds, and multiply by 4 to estimate the beats per minute.

Use: Common in basic health checks and physical exams.

**The 300 Method:**

Method: On an EKG strip, identify a QRS complex that lines up with a heavy line on the paper. Count the number of large squares between that QRS complex and the next, and divide 300 by this number.

Use: Effective for regular rhythms.

**The 1500 Method:**

Method: Count the number of small squares between two successive QRS complexes and divide 1500 by this number.

Use: Offers more precision, especially suitable for irregular rhythms.

EKG Interpretation - Sequence Method:

Method: This involves using a pre-calculated sequence (300, 150, 100, 75, 60, 50) based on the large squares on an EKG strip. The number 300 represents one large square, 150 for two, and so on. Align a QRS complex with a heavy line and move to the next QRS complex along this sequence to estimate the rate.

Use: Quick and practical for both regular and slightly irregular rhythms.

**Electronic Monitors:**

Method: Devices like EKG machines, smartwatches, and fitness trackers automatically calculate the heart rate using electronic sensors.

Use: Convenient for continuous monitoring of heart rate, especially during physical activity or throughout the day.

**Normal Heartbeat**
**PR** =0.20 sec
**QRS**=0.04 sec
**QT**=0.40 se

# VI. EKG STRIP ANALYSIS

1.  Reading 2-Lead Strips
2.  Interpretation Techniques
3.  Axis Determination

## 1-Basics of 2-Strips in EKG

The concept of "2-Strips" in EKG (Electrocardiogram) refers to a brief, focused recording of the heart's electrical activity using two leads, typically over a short duration like a 6-second interval. This method is often used for a quick assessment of cardiac rhythm and heart rate. Here's an explanation of the basics of 2-Strip EKG:

### Purpose and Use:

Rapid Assessment: 2-Strips are primarily used for quick evaluations, especially in settings where a full 12-lead EKG is not necessary or feasible.

Monitoring: They are useful in continuous monitoring settings, such as in hospitals where patients require regular but brief cardiac check-ups.

### Lead Selection:

Common Leads: The most used leads for 2-Strips are Lead II (for a clear view of the P wave and rhythm) and either Lead V1 or Lead V5 (for a better view of the QRS complex and T wave).

Lead Placement: Lead II is placed across the heart (right arm to left leg), while Lead V1 or V5 is placed on the chest.

### Interpreting a 2-Strip EKG:

Heart Rhythm: One of the primary purposes of a 2-Strip is to assess the regularity and type of heart rhythm (e.g., sinus rhythm, atrial fibrillation, or other arrhythmias).

Heart Rate: It allows for a quick calculation of heart rate by counting the number of QRS complexes in the 6-second strip and multiplying by 10.

Identifying Abnormalities: While limited, 2-Strips can help identify significant abnormalities in the heart's rhythm that may require further investigation.

### Limitations:

Limited View: Since only two leads are used, 2-Strips provide a limited view of the heart's electrical activity. They are not as comprehensive as a 12-lead EKG.

Potential for Missed Diagnoses: Certain cardiac conditions that are better identified with other leads may be missed on a 2-Strip.

### Clinical Application:

ER and ICU Use: Frequently used in emergency rooms and intensive care units for quick assessments.

Ambulatory and Outpatient Settings: Useful for rapid checks in ambulatory care or during routine physical examinations.

In summary, 2-Strip EKGs are a valuable tool in various clinical settings for rapid assessment of cardiac rhythm and rate, offering a balance between efficiency and diagnostic insight. However, they are not a substitute for a full 12-lead EKG when comprehensive cardiac evaluation is needed.

## 2. Interpretation Techniques

### Rhythm Definition and Importance

Definition: In an EKG, 'rhythm' refers to the pattern of electrical activity of the heart as represented by the P waves, QRS complexes, and T waves. It indicates how regularly the heart beats and where the electrical impulses originate.

Importance: Understanding rhythm is crucial because it reveals the health and functionality of the heart's electrical system. Abnormal rhythms can indicate various cardiac conditions like arrhythmias (irregular heartbeat), ischemia (reduced blood flow), or structural heart problems.

### Rhythm Regularity:
Rhythm regularity refers to the consistency of intervals between heartbeats. Analyzing rhythm regularity is crucial in EKG interpretation, as it helps identify various cardiac arrhythmias and assess heart health.

### Assessing Rhythm Regularity
### Regular Rhythms:
The intervals between successive heartbeats are consistent.

Common regular rhythms include normal sinus rhythm, sinus tachycardia, and sinus bradycardia.

### Irregular Rhythms:
The intervals between heartbeats vary.

Types include regularly irregular (consistent pattern of irregularity, like in atrial flutter with variable block) and irregularly irregular (no consistent pattern, as in atrial fibrillation).

### Assessment Techniques:
Visual Inspection: Observing the consistency of intervals between P waves (atrial rhythm) and QRS complexes (ventricular rhythm) on an EKG strip.

Paper Method: Marking the R waves on a paper strip and moving it along the EKG to see if the R-R intervals match up consistently.

## Using a Caliper in EKG
Calipers are precision tools used in EKG interpretation to measure intervals and assess rhythm regularity.

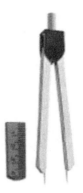

## How to Use a Caliper
### Setting the Caliper:
Adjust the caliper so that its points align with two consecutive R waves (R-R interval) or P waves (P-P interval).

Checking Regularity:
Move the caliper along the EKG strip, keeping one point fixed on an R wave while moving the other to the next R wave.
A regular rhythm will have the caliper's points consistently aligning with each R wave.

Measuring Intervals:
Use the caliper to measure other intervals like the PR interval or QT interval. Align the caliper's points with the beginning and end of the interval and compare it to the EKG's scale.

Identifying Irregularities:

Variations in the distances between caliper points when moved along the strip indicate irregular rhythms.

### Tips for Using Calipers

Accuracy: Ensure the caliper is precisely aligned with the EKG markings for accurate measurements.

Steady Hand: Keep a steady hand to avoid small movements that can lead to inaccurate readings.

Cross-Check: Use the caliper in conjunction with other methods (like the 300 method for rate calculation) for a comprehensive analysis.

Calipers are particularly useful in distinguishing between different types of arrhythmias based on the regularity and measurement of intervals, and they enhance the precision of EKG interpretation.

### P Wave Analysis:

**Significance**: P waves represent atrial depolarization. Consistent P waves preceding each QRS complex suggest a sinus rhythm originating from the SA node.

**Abnormalities:** Absent, irregular, or abnormal P waves can indicate atrial fibrillation, atrial flutter, or other atrial arrhythmias.

### QRS Complex Evaluation:

**Width and Shape**: A normal QRS complex duration is 0.06 to 0.10 seconds. Wider complexes may indicate ventricular rhythms or conduction blocks.

**Orientation**: The direction of the QRS complex (positive or negative) in different leads helps in identifying the site of rhythm origin.

### Identifying Patterns:

**Specific Rhythms**: Patterns like regular, rapid QRS complexes may suggest ventricular tachycardia; irregularly irregular rhythm with no distinct P waves may indicate atrial fibrillation.

## 3. Axis Determination Methods

### Quadrant Method:

Leads I and aVF: Look at the QRS complex in leads I and aVF. If the QRS complex is positive in both leads, the axis is normal. Variations can indicate left or right axis deviation.

### Isoelectric Lead Method:

Finding the Isoelectric Lead: Identify the lead where the QRS complex has equal upward and downward deflections. The perpendicular lead gives the heart's electrical axis.

### Hex axial Reference System:

Six-Limb Leads: Uses leads I, II, III, aVR, aVL, and aVF to precisely determine the axis. By finding the lead with the most positive QRS complex, the axis can be pinpointed on the hex axial reference system.

Normal Axis: Typically falls between -30° and +90°.

# VII-RHYTHM NOMENCLATURE

## 1-Definition of Rhythm

In the context of cardiac health and physiology, "rhythm" refers to the pattern of electrical impulses that coordinate the heart's contractions. It is the sequence and regularity of heartbeats, which are crucial for maintaining effective and efficient blood circulation.

Key Aspects of Heart Rhythm
1.   Origin: Normally, the heart rhythm is initiated by the sinoatrial (SA) node, the natural pacemaker of the heart, located in the right atrium.
2.   Rate: This is the number of heartbeats per minute. A normal resting heart rate for adults typically ranges from 60 to 100 beats per minute.
3.   Regularity: Refers to the consistency of the intervals between heartbeats. In a regular rhythm, these intervals are uniform.
4.   Sequence of Cardiac Events: Includes the depolarization and repolarization of atria and ventricles, which is crucial for effective blood pumping.

## 2-Normal Sinus Rhythm (NSR)

**Characteristics:** A heart rate of 60-100 bpm, with each P wave followed by a QRS complex and T wave. The rhythm is regular, and the P wave is upright in leads I and II, indicating normal atrial depolarization.

**Clinical Significance:** NSR is considered the normal heart rhythm; deviations from this pattern often indicate underlying cardiac or systemic issues.

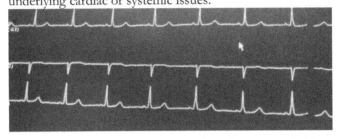

## Variants of Sinus Rhythms
## 3. Sinus Tachycardia and Sinus Bradycardia

### Sinus Tachycardia:
Rate: Faster than 100 bpm, but less than 180 bpm.

Causes: Can be physiological (exercise, stress) or pathological (fever, anemia, heart failure).

ECG Features: Similar to NSR but with a faster rate.

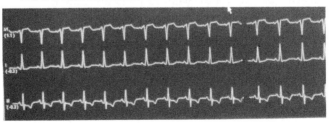

### Sinus Bradycardia:
Rate: Slower than 60 bpm.

Causes: Common in athletes, during sleep, or as a result of vagal stimulation, hypothyroidism, or certain medications.

ECG Features: Similar to NSR but with a slower rate.

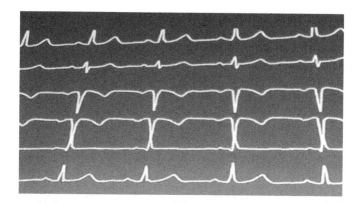

## 4. Sinus Arrhythmia:

Sinus Arrhythmia is a variation of the normal heartbeat, which is characterized by slight changes in the heart rate during the breathing cycle. It is typically considered a benign condition, especially common in children and young adults.

### Characteristics

**Rhythm**: The rhythm of a sinus arrhythmia is generally regular, but it varies with respiration. The heart rate increases slightly during inhalation (inspiration) and decreases during exhalation (expiration).

**Heart Rate**: While the heart rate may fluctuate, it usually stays within the normal range for age.

**ECG Findings:** On an ECG, sinus arrhythmia is characterized by a slight variation in the R-R intervals, which are the intervals between consecutive QRS complexes. The P waves are normal and upright in leads I and II, and each P wave is followed by a normal QRS complex.

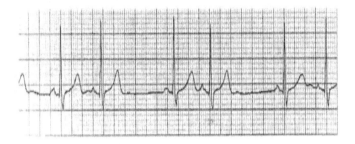

## 5. Sinus Arrest or Pause

Sinus arrest or sinus pause is a cardiac rhythm disturbance characterized by a temporary interruption in the normal pace making activity of the sinoatrial (SA) node, the heart's primary pacemaker. This interruption results in a transient absence of electrical activity and, consequently, a missed or delayed heartbeat.

### Characteristics
**ECG Findings**: On an electrocardiogram (ECG), sinus arrest is identified by a sudden and unexpected absence of P waves for a duration that is longer than the normal P-P interval. This pause is followed by the resumption of normal P waves and QRS complexes.

**Heart Rate and Rhythm**: During a sinus arrest, the heart rate drops during the pause and resumes its normal pace post-pause. The rhythm is generally regular, except for the pause.

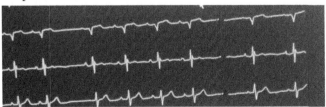

## 6. Sick Sinus Syndrome (SSS)

Sick Sinus Syndrome, also known as Sinus Node Dysfunction, is a group of heart rhythm disorders that occur when the sinoatrial (SA) node, the heart's natural pacemaker, does not function properly. This condition is most common in older adults and can lead to a variety of heart rhythm complications.

### Characteristics of SSS

Variable Rhythms: SSS can manifest as bradycardia (slow heart rate), tachycardia (fast heart rate), or a combination of both (tachy-brady syndrome).

**ECG Findings**: The electrocardiogram may show sinus bradycardia, sinus arrest, or pause. In tachy-brady syndrome, periods of rapid heart rates (like atrial fibrillation) alternate with slow rates.

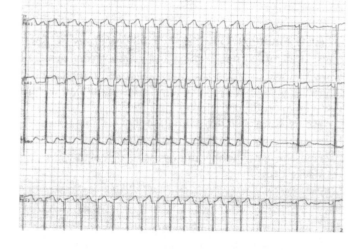

# VIII. PREMATURE BEATS AND ECTOPIC RHYTHMS

1. Premature Atrial, Ventricular, and Junctional Contractions
2. Escape Beats: Atrial and Ventricular

## 1. Premature Beats

### Premature Atrial Contractions (PACs)

Premature Atrial Contractions (PACs) are early heartbeats that originate from the atria, the upper chambers of the heart. They are common cardiac arrhythmias and can occur in healthy individuals as well as those with heart disease.

#### Characteristics

**ECG Findings: Early P Wave**: PACs are characterized by an early P wave that has a different morphology compared to the P waves originating from the sinoatrial (SA) node. This P wave is often followed by a QRS complex.

**Compensatory Pause**: After the PAC, there is typically a compensatory pause, meaning the next normal heartbeat may appear later than expected, as the heart resets its rhythm.

**Heart Rhythm: Despite** the premature beat, the underlying heart rhythm is usually normal (e.g., sinus rhythm).

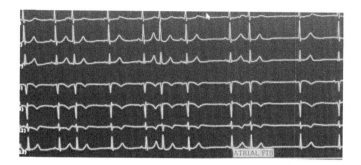

## Atrial Arrhythmias
### Atrial Couplet

**Definition**: An atrial couplet consists of two consecutive premature atrial contractions (PACs).

**ECG Characteristics**: On an ECG, an atrial couplet is seen as two early P waves followed by their respective QRS complexes. These P waves often have a different morphology compared to the normal P waves because they originate from a different part of the atria.

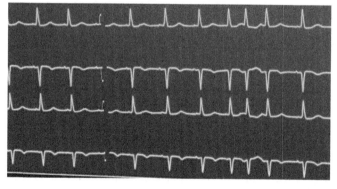

### Atrial Triplet

**Definition**: This refers to three consecutive PACs.

**ECG Characteristics**: Similar to couplets, triplets will show three aberrant P waves, each followed by a QRS complex, occurring earlier than the expected sinus rhythm.

**Clinical Consideration**: Atrial triplets can be a precursor to more sustained forms of atrial tachycardia, including atrial flutter or atrial fibrillation.

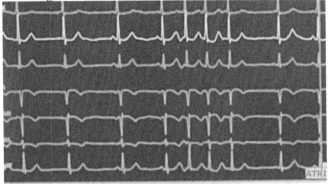

### Atrial Bigeminy

**Definition**: Atrial bigeminy occurs when a normal beat is followed by a PAC, and this pattern repeats consistently – one normal beat followed by one premature beat.

**ECG Characteristics**: You'll see a regular alternation of a normal P-QRS-T cycle and an early P-QRS sequence. The premature P wave typically looks different from the normal P wave.

**Clinical Significance**: This pattern can be intermittent and might be triggered by factors like caffeine, alcohol, or stress. Persistent bigeminy may need further assessment to rule out underlying heart conditions.

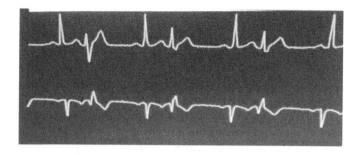

### Atrial Trigeminy

**Definition**: In atrial trigeminy, two normal heartbeats are followed by a PAC, and this three-beat pattern repeats consistently.

**ECG Characteristics**: The ECG will show two normal sinus beats followed by an early and aberrant atrial contraction.

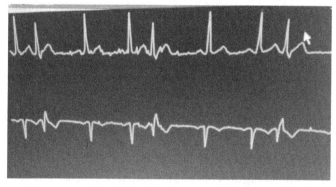

### Premature Ventricular Contractions (PVCs)

Premature Ventricular Contractions (PVCs) are early heartbeats that originate from the ventricles, the lower chambers of the heart. They are among the most common types of cardiac arrhythmias and can occur in both healthy individuals and those with heart disease.

**Characteristics**

**ECG Findings: Wide and Bizarre QRS**: PVCs are identified on an ECG by a wide and bizarre QRS complex, typically lasting longer than 0.12 seconds. The QRS complexes of PVCs look different from the normal QRS complexes because they are not originating from the usual conduction pathway.

**No Preceding P Wave:** There is typically no preceding P wave, or the P wave may occur just after the QRS complex.

**Compensatory Pause**: Often, PVCs are followed by a compensatory pause – the heart "resets," causing a pause before the next regular heartbeat.

**Heart Rhythm**: The underlying rhythm can be any rhythm, but PVCs interrupt it with their premature beats.

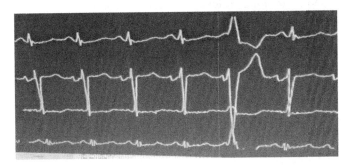

**Ventricular Arrhythmias: Couplets, Triplets, Bigeminy, and Trigeminy**

Ventricular arrhythmias, including couplets, triplets, bigeminy, and trigeminy, involve abnormal heartbeats originating from the ventricles. These are often more concerning than atrial arrhythmias due to the ventricles' critical role in pumping blood throughout the body.

**Ventricular Couplet**

Definition: A ventricular couplet consists of two consecutive premature ventricular contractions (PVCs).

ECG Characteristics: On an ECG, a ventricular couplet appears as two wide and bizarre QRS complexes, occurring earlier than expected, with no preceding P waves.

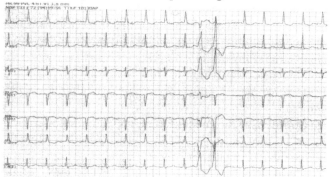

### Ventricular Triplet

Definition: Three consecutive PVCs form a ventricular triplet.

ECG Characteristics: Similar to couplets, triplets are identified on ECG as three successive wide, early QRS complexes.

Clinical Consideration: Triplet PVCs are concerning as they may progress to ventricular tachycardia, especially in patients with underlying heart conditions.

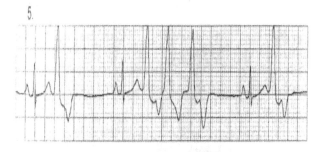

### Ventricular Bigeminy

Definition: In ventricular bigeminy, every normal beat is followed by a PVC. This pattern of one normal beat alternating with one premature beat continues consistently.

ECG Characteristics: Regular alternation of a normal QRS complex and a wide, premature QRS complex. The premature beats have a different morphology from the normal beats.

Clinical Relevance: Bigeminy can occur intermittently and might be benign in some cases, but persistent bigeminy, especially in heart disease patients, requires careful evaluation and management.

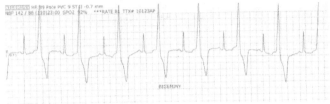

### Ventricular Trigeminy

Definition: Ventricular trigeminy occurs when two normal heartbeats are followed by a PVC in a repeating three-beat pattern.

ECG Characteristics: Two normal sinus beats followed by an early, wide QRS complex.

Clinical Implication: Like bigeminy, trigeminy can be benign or a sign of an underlying condition. Persistent or symptomatic trigeminy warrants further investigation.

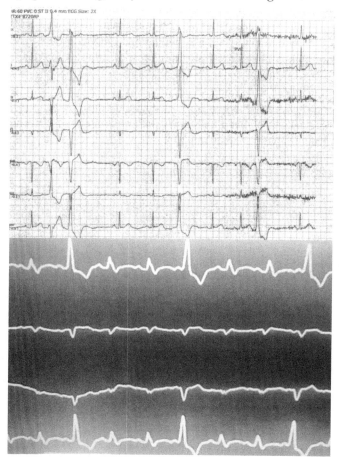

**Multifocal PVCs (Premature Ventricular Contractions)**

Definition

Multifocal PVCs are premature ventricular contractions arising from different locations within the ventricles. This results in PVCs with varying morphologies (shapes) on an electrocardiogram (ECG).

ECG Characteristics

Varying QRS Morphologies: The most distinguishing feature of multifocal PVCs is the presence of multiple different QRS complex shapes within the same ECG tracing.

Premature Occurrence: PVCs occur earlier than the expected normal beat.

Compensatory Pause: Often followed by a compensatory pause – a longer interval before the next normal heartbeat.

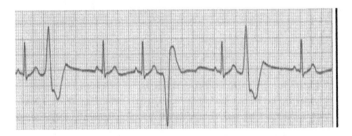

## Premature Junctional Contractions (PJCs)

Premature Junctional Contractions (PJCs) are a type of arrhythmia where the heartbeat originates prematurely from the atrioventricular (AV) junctional tissue, the area around the AV node which lies at the boundary between the atria and ventricles.

### Characteristics

ECG Findings:

Narrow QRS Complexes: PJCs typically produce a narrow QRS complex, similar to a normal heartbeat, because the ventricles are activated in the usual manner through the His-Purkinje system.

Absent or Inverted P Waves: The P wave may be absent, or if present, it may appear just before, during, or after the

QRS complex. When occurring before the QRS complex, P waves are often inverted due to retrograde conduction.

Compensatory Pause: Often, PJCs are followed by a compensatory pause, as the next normal sinus beat comes a little later than expected.

Rhythm:

The underlying rhythm can be regular, but the presence of PJCs interrupts this regularity.

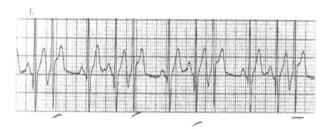

### Ectopy: Detailed Explanation
Definition

Ectopy refers to a cardiac event where an electrical impulse originates from a site other than the sinoatrial (SA) node, the heart's natural pacemaker. This abnormal impulse generation leads to **premature heartbeats or arrhythmias.**

### Types of Ectopy
Atrial Ectopy:

Originates from an ectopic focus within the atria.

Results in premature atrial contractions (PACs) or atrial tachyarrhythmias like atrial fibrillation or flutter.

### Ventricular Ectopy:
Occurs when the impulse originates in the ventricles.

Leads to premature ventricular contractions (PVCs) or ventricular tachycardia (VT).

### Junctional Ectopy:
Arises from the atrioventricular (AV) junction.

Can cause junctional premature beats or junctional tachycardia.

ECG Characteristics

Premature Beats: Ectopic beats occur earlier than the next expected normal beat.

Abnormal Waveform: The morphology of ectopic beats differs from normal sinus beats. In atrial ectopy, abnormal P waves are observed; in ventricular ectopy, wide and bizarre QRS complexes are seen.

Compensatory Pause: Often follows ectopic beats, especially PVCs, due to the resetting of the heart's electrical rhythm.

Clinical Significance

Symptoms: Can range from being asymptomatic to causing palpitations, dizziness, or even syncope.

Risk Assessment: Frequent or complex ectopic beats (like runs of VT or multifocal PVCs) in patients with heart disease can signify a higher risk of more serious arrhythmias.

Causes

Cardiac Conditions: Underlying heart disease, myocardial infarction, cardiomyopathies, or structural abnormalities.

Electrolyte Imbalances: Especially abnormalities in potassium, magnesium, or calcium.

Stimulants: Such as caffeine, alcohol, nicotine, and certain medications.

Stress and Anxiety: Psychological factors can exacerbate ectopic activity.

Management

Lifestyle Modifications: Reducing caffeine intake, stress management, and smoking cessation.

Medication Review: Adjusting or discontinuing medications that may contribute to ectopy.

Treating Underlying Conditions: Managing any heart conditions or electrolyte imbalances.

Monitoring: Regular follow-up, especially in patients with heart disease, is important.

Pharmacological Treatment: Beta-blockers, calcium channel blockers, or other antiarrhythmic drugs may be used in symptomatic cases or if there is an associated risk of more serious arrhythmias.

Prognosis

The impact of ectopy largely depends on the underlying heart health and the type and frequency of ectopic beats. In individuals with a healthy heart, isolated ectopic beats are generally benign, but in the context of heart disease, they may require more careful management.

Summary

Ectopy represents an abnormal origin of cardiac electrical impulses leading to premature beats or arrhythmias. Its significance varies based on the individual's overall cardiac health and the presence of other risk factors. Management strategies are tailored to the underlying cause and the frequency and type of ectopic activity. Regular monitoring and addressing modifiable risk factors are key to managing ectopic beats.

## 2. Escape Beats

Escape beats are heartbeats that occur when the heart's primary pacemaker (the sinoatrial, or SA, node) fails to initiate a beat, or its impulse is blocked. Secondary pacemakers within the heart then "escape" the control of the SA node and generate a compensatory beat. These secondary pacemakers can be located in the atria, the AV junction, or the ventricles.

### Atrial Escape Beats

Origin: Arise from an ectopic focus within the atria, outside the SA node.

ECG Characteristics: Characterized by an abnormal P wave with a different morphology from the sinus P wave, followed by a normal QRS complex. The atrial escape beat occurs later than the expected sinus beat.

Clinical Significance: Atrial escape beats are generally benign and often occur when the sinus rate is slow, allowing an ectopic atrial focus to take over temporarily.

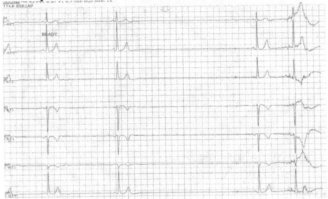

### Ventricular Escape Beats

Origin: Originate in the ventricular myocardium.

ECG Characteristics: Present as a wide and bizarre QRS complex, occurring after a significant pause in the heart's rhythm. There is no preceding P wave, or it may occur just after the QRS complex.

Clinical Significance: Ventricular escape beats can be seen in conditions of severe bradycardia or AV block, where the higher pacemaking sites (SA node or AV junction) fail to maintain an adequate heart rate. They are crucial for maintaining a minimal level of cardiac output in such situations but can indicate significant underlying heart disease.

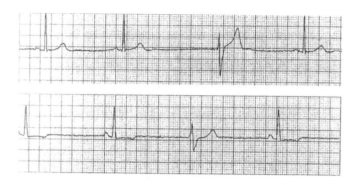

### Junctional Escape Beats

Origin: Arise from the AV junctional tissue.

ECG Characteristics: Typically exhibit a narrow QRS complex, similar to a normal heartbeat. The P wave may be absent, inverted, or occur just after the QRS complex. They emerge after a pause and are often slower than the intrinsic rate of the SA node.

Clinical Significance: Junctional escape beats usually occur when the heart rate is very slow, and like ventricular escape beats, they serve as a protective mechanism against excessive bradycardia. They can indicate dysfunction of the SA node or a block in the atrial-to-ventricular conduction pathway.

17.

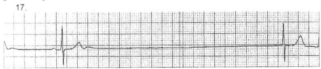

# IX-COMPLEX ATRIAL AND JUNCTIONAL RHYTHMS

1. Atrial Tachycardia and its Types
2. Supraventricular Tachycardia (SVT)
3. Wolf-Parkinson-White Syndrome
4. Atrial Fibrillation and Flutter
5. Junctional Rhythms and Variants

## 1-Atrial Tachycardia and its Types

Atrial Tachycardia (AT) is a type of supraventricular tachycardia characterized by a rapid heart rhythm originating from the atria, the upper chambers of the heart. The atrial rate in AT typically ranges from **100 to 250 beats per minute**.

Characteristics of Atrial Tachycardia

ECG Findings: The ECG typically shows a rapid, regular series of distinct P waves with an abnormal morphology, followed by normal QRS complexes. The P wave morphology in AT differs from that seen in normal sinus rhythm due to the abnormal origin of the atrial impulse.

Mechanism: It results from an abnormal focus or circuit within the atria that takes over the heart's rhythm, bypassing the normal pacemaking function of the sinoatrial (SA) node.

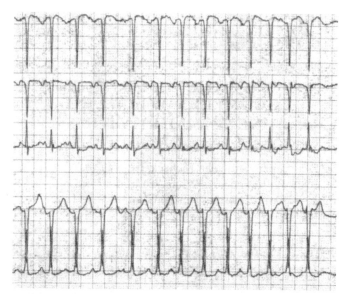

## Types of Atrial Tachycardia
## Focal Atrial Tachycardia:

Origin: Arises from a single ectopic focus within the atria.

ECG Features: Consistent P wave morphology, as all beats originate from the same location.

Triggers: Can be triggered by stress, caffeine, or structural heart disease.

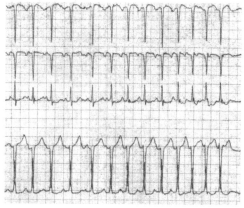

## Multifocal Atrial Tachycardia (MAT):

Characteristics: Multiple ectopic foci within the atria generate impulses, leading to a chaotic rhythm.

ECG Features: Varying P wave morphologies and irregular P-P intervals.

Associated Conditions: Often seen in patients with severe pulmonary diseases, such as chronic obstructive pulmonary disease (COPD).

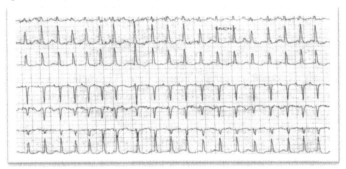

## Paroxysmal Atrial Tachycardia (PAT):

Features: Sudden onset and termination of rapid, regular atrial contractions.

ECG Characteristics: A series of rapid P waves with a consistent morphology, followed by normal QRS complexes.

Symptoms: Can include palpitations, dizziness, or chest discomfort.

Clinical Significance

Symptoms: Symptoms of AT can range from palpitations and shortness of breath to more severe effects like chest pain or syncope, depending on the rate and the individual's cardiac function.

Risk Factors: While it can occur in individuals without heart disease, it's more common in those with underlying cardiac conditions, electrolyte imbalances, or after heart surgery.

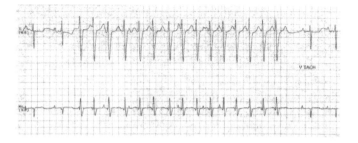

## 2-Supraventricular Tachycardia (SVT)

Supraventricular Tachycardia (SVT) is a broad term encompassing various tachyarrhythmias (fast heart rhythms) that originate above the ventricles, typically involving the atria or the atrioventricular (AV) junction.

Characteristics of SVT

Heart Rate: SVT usually presents with a rapid heart rate, often ranging from **150 to 220 beats per minute.**

ECG Findings: Characterized by narrow QRS complexes (unless there is an existing bundle branch block or rate-related aberrancy), often with a regular rhythm. P waves may be difficult to discern and can be hidden within or occur just after the QRS complex.

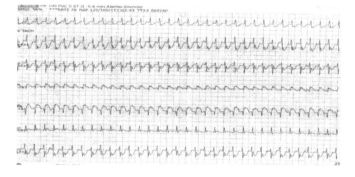

Types of SVT

## Atrioventricular Nodal Reentrant Tachycardia (AVNRT):

Most common form of SVT.

Involves a reentrant circuit within or near the AV node.

Typically presents with sudden onset and termination.

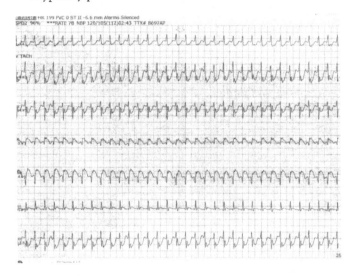

## Atrioventricular Reentrant Tachycardia (AVRT):

Associated with an accessory pathway, like in Wolff-Parkinson-White syndrome.

Can involve reentrant circuits passing through the accessory pathway.

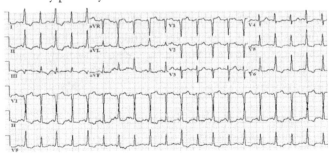

**Atrial Tachycardia:**
Originates from an ectopic focus within the atria.
Can be focal or multifocal.
Clinical Presentation
Symptoms: Palpitations, dizziness, chest discomfort, shortness of breath, or in severe cases, syncope (fainting).
Onset: SVT can have a sudden onset, often triggered by stress, caffeine, alcohol, or exercise.

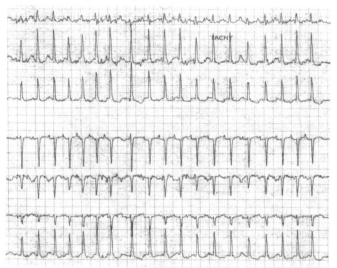

## Differences Between Supraventricular Tachycardia (SVT) and Atrial Tachycardia (AT) with an Emphasis on Heart Rate

Supraventricular Tachycardia (SVT) and Atrial Tachycardia (AT) are both types of arrhythmias originating from above the ventricles. While they share some similarities, there are distinct differences, particularly in their mechanisms, heart rate characteristics, and ECG presentations.

### Supraventricular Tachycardia (SVT)
**Broad Classification:** SVT is a general term that encompasses various tachyarrhythmias originating from the

atria or the AV node. It includes conditions such as Atrioventricular Nodal Reentrant Tachycardia (AVNRT), Atrioventricular Reentrant Tachycardia (AVRT), and AT.

**Heart Rate:** SVT typically presents with a rapid heart rate, usually between 150 to 220 beats per minute. The rate is often very consistent and regular.

**ECG Characteristics**: The ECG in SVT generally shows a regular, narrow QRS complex tachycardia. The P wave is often not visible, merged within the QRS complex, or occurs just after the QRS complex.

Onset and Termination: Episodes of SVT frequently start and stop suddenly ("paroxysmal").

### Atrial Tachycardia (AT)

**Specific Type of SVT:** AT is a specific type of SVT that originates from an ectopic focus within the atria, outside of the SA node.

**Heart Rate:** In AT, the heart rate is usually somewhat slower than in other types of SVT, typically ranging from 100 to 200 beats per minute. The rate can be regular or slightly irregular.

**ECG Characteristics**: AT is characterized by abnormal P waves with a different morphology from those of sinus rhythm, followed by normal QRS complexes. The P waves in AT are distinct and usually visible on the ECG.

Onset and Termination: AT may start and stop more gradually compared to other forms of SVT.

### Key Differences

Heart Rate:

SVT tends to have a higher heart rate (150-220 bpm), with a very regular rhythm.

AT usually presents with a slightly lower heart rate (100-200 bpm) and can have a regular or slightly irregular rhythm.

### Origin and Mechanism:

SVT involves various mechanisms, including reentrant circuits around the AV node or involving accessory pathways.

AT arises from an ectopic atrial focus, independent of the AV node.

### ECG Presentation:

In typical SVT forms like AVNRT, the P wave is often hidden or difficult to discern.

In AT, the P wave is more prominent and has an abnormal morphology compared to normal sinus rhythm.

### Clinical Features:

SVT episodes often have a sudden onset and termination.

AT may be more persistent and less paroxysmal in nature.

Understanding these differences is critical for accurate diagnosis and appropriate management of these arrhythmias. While both SVT and AT present with rapid heart rates, their specific rates, ECG characteristics, and response to treatment vary, guiding the therapeutic approach.

## 3-Wolf-Parkinson-White Syndrome (WPW)

Wolf-Parkinson-White Syndrome is a specific type of supraventricular tachycardia (SVT) characterized by an abnormal additional electrical pathway (accessory pathway) between the atria and ventricles. This condition is congenital (present at birth) and is one of the most common causes of fast heart rate disorders in infants and children.

### Characteristics of WPW

Abnormal Pathway: The key feature of WPW is the presence of an extra pathway (known as the Bundle of Kent) that bypasses the normal route through the atrioventricular (AV) node. This pathway allows electrical signals to pass directly from the atria to the ventricles, potentially leading to rapid heart rates.

### ECG Findings:

Delta Wave: A classic sign of WPW on an ECG is the presence of a "delta wave," which is a slurred upstroke in the QRS complex, resulting from the early activation of the ventricles via the accessory pathway.

Short PR Interval: The time between the onset of the P wave and the start of the QRS complex (PR interval) is shortened.

Wide QRS Complex: The QRS complex is often wider than normal due to the abnormal conduction pathway.

### Clinical Presentation

Symptoms: Can include palpitations, dizziness, shortness of breath, chest pain, and in severe cases, syncope (fainting). In some individuals, WPW may be asymptomatic and discovered incidentally during an ECG.

Arrhythmias: People with WPW are at risk of developing rapid heart rate conditions, including atrial fibrillation, atrial flutter, and other forms of SVT.

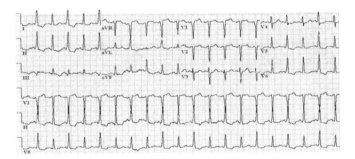

## 4-Atrial Fibrillation and Aflutter (AF)

Atrial Fibrillation is the most common type of serious arrhythmia. It's characterized by rapid and irregular beating of the atrial chambers of the heart.

Characteristics

Rapid and Irregular Rhythm: The atria beat chaotically and irregularly, out of coordination with the ventricles.

ECG Findings: Characterized by an irregularly irregular rhythm, absence of distinct P waves, and irregular QRS intervals. The atrial activity is instead replaced by rapid oscillations or fibrillatory waves.

Causes

Common in Older Adults: The risk increases with age.

Heart Disease: Often seen in individuals with underlying heart diseases such as hypertension, coronary artery disease, and heart failure.

Other Factors: Can occur due to other factors like hyperthyroidism, acute alcohol intoxication ("holiday heart syndrome"), or pulmonary embolism.

Clinical Significance

Stroke Risk: AF can lead to blood clots in the heart, which can travel to the brain, causing a stroke.

Heart Failure: The irregular and fast rhythm can weaken the heart, leading to heart failure.

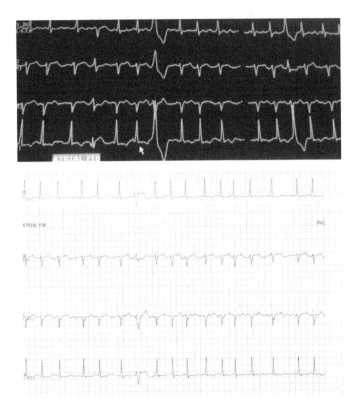

## Rapid Atrial Fibrillation

Rapid Atrial Fibrillation (often abbreviated as "Rapid AF" or "Rapid AFib") refers to a form of atrial fibrillation where the heart rate, specifically in the ventricles, is significantly faster than normal. This rapid rate is due to the irregular and chaotic atrial activity characteristic of AFib, which leads to an irregularly irregular and often rapid response in the ventricles.

Characteristics

Heart Rate: In rapid AFib, the ventricular rate often exceeds 100 beats per minute and can sometimes reach 150-180 beats per minute or higher.

ECG Findings: The electrocardiogram (ECG) in rapid AFib shows an irregularly irregular rhythm with no discernible P waves. The QRS complexes, which represent ventricular contraction, vary in timing (R-R intervals) and can be normal or wide if there is an underlying conduction delay or aberrancy.

## Pathophysiology

In atrial fibrillation, the atria (upper chambers of the heart) fibrillate, or quiver, due to multiple erratic electrical impulses. These impulses are conducted irregularly to the ventricles through the atrioventricular (AV) node.

The rapidity of the ventricular response in AFib depends on the AV node's refractory period – the shorter this period, the more impulses are conducted, leading to a faster heart rate.

## Symptoms and Clinical Significance

Symptoms: Can include palpitations, shortness of breath, fatigue, dizziness, or chest discomfort. In extreme cases, it can lead to syncope (fainting).

Risks: Rapid AFib increases the risk of developing heart failure due to the sustained fast heart rate, which can impair the heart's ability to pump efficiently. There is also an increased risk of stroke.

Complications: If left untreated, rapid AFib can lead to tachycardia-induced cardiomyopathy, a condition where the persistent high heart rate weakens the heart muscle.

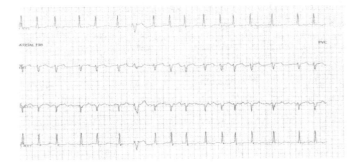

## Atrial Flutter

Atrial Flutter is less common than AF but shares some similarities. It's characterized by a rapid and regular rhythm originating from the atria.

Characteristics

Circuit in the Atria: Involves a single electrical circuit looping through the atrium, typically at a rate of about 300 beats per minute.

ECG Findings: Shows a **"sawtooth" pattern**, particularly visible in leads II, III, and aVF, due to the regular atrial activity.

Causes and Risks

Similar to AF, it can be associated with heart disease, surgery, or lung disease.

### Clinical Significance

Symptoms: Can include palpitations, shortness of breath, and fatigue.

**Complications**: Risk of stroke and heart failure, similar to AF.

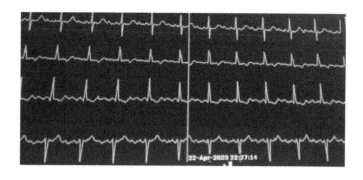

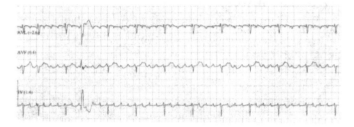

## 5-Junctional Rhythms and Variants

Junctional rhythms are cardiac arrhythmias that originate from the atrioventricular (AV) junction, which includes the AV node and the area surrounding it. These rhythms can occur when the sinoatrial (SA) node's activity is suppressed or its impulse conduction to the rest of the heart is impaired.

### Characteristics of Junctional Rhythms

Origin: Arise from the cells in the AV junction, which have an intrinsic pacing capability, though typically slower than the SA node.

**ECG Findings:** Characterized by narrow QRS complexes. The P waves may be absent, inverted, or occur just before or after the QRS complex, depending on the site of origin within the AV junction.

### Types of Junctional Rhythms
### Junctional Escape Rhythm:

Rate: Typically **40-60 beats per minute**.

Mechanism: Occurs when the rate of the SA node falls below the intrinsic rate of the AV junction.

ECG Features: Narrow QRS complexes with a regular rhythm; P waves may be inverted or absent.

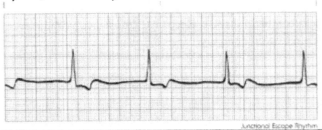

Junctional Escape Rhythm

### Accelerated Junctional Rhythm:

Rate: Faster than a typical junctional escape rhythm, usually **60-100 beats per minute.**

Mechanism: Enhanced automaticity in the AV junction, often due to conditions like digitalis toxicity, ischemia, or post-surgical intervention.

ECG Features: Similar to junctional escape rhythm but with a faster rate.

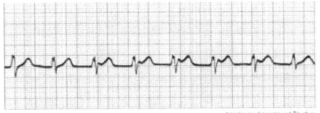

Accelerated Junctional Rhythm

### Junctional Tachycardia:

Rate: Exceeds 100 beats per minute, can reach up to **150-180 bpm.**

Mechanism: Usually due to increased automaticity or reentry within the AV junction.

ECG Features: Rapid, regular narrow QRS complexes, often with hidden or inverted P waves.

Clinical Significance

Symptoms: Junctional rhythms can be asymptomatic, especially if the rate is not too fast or too slow. Symptoms, when present, may include palpitations, lightheadedness, or dizziness.

Risk Factors: Can be seen in various conditions, including heart disease, electrolyte imbalances, drug effects, or after cardiac surgery.

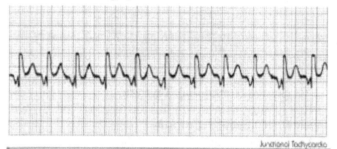

Junctional Tachycardia

# X-HEART BLOCKS

1. Different Degrees of AV Blocks
2. AV Dissociation and its Implications
3. Bundle Branch Block and its Types
4. Blocked PAC

## 1-Different Degrees of AV Blocks

Atrioventricular (AV) blocks are a type of heart block characterized by a delay or interruption in the electrical signal from the atria to the ventricles. They are classified into three main degrees, each with distinct features and clinical implications.

### First-Degree AV Block

Description: A consistent delay in the conduction from the atria to the ventricles.

ECG Findings:

Prolonged PR interval (greater than 0.20 seconds).

Each P wave is followed by a QRS complex.

### Clinical Significance:

Often asymptomatic and may be found in healthy individuals, especially athletes.

Can be associated with certain medications or myocardial ischemia.

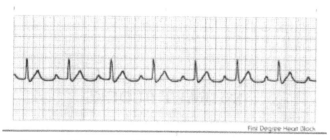

First Degree Heart Block

## Second-Degree AV Block: Type I (Mobitz I/Wenckebach)

Overview

Type I Second-Degree AV Block, also known as Mobitz I or Wenckebach block, is characterized by progressive lengthening of the atrioventricular (AV) conduction time (PR interval on the ECG) until a beat is 'dropped' – an atrial impulse fails to conduct to the ventricles, resulting in a missed QRS complex.

ECG Characteristics

Progressive PR Interval Lengthening: The hallmark of Wenckebach block is the gradual prolongation of the PR interval with each successive heartbeat.

Pattern of Conduction and Non-conduction: After several beats with lengthening PR intervals, there is a non-conducted P wave (a 'dropped' beat), after which the cycle restarts.

Normal or Slightly Slow Heart Rate: The overall heart rate is often normal or slightly bradycardic.

Clinical Presentation

Often asymptomatic, particularly in young and healthy individuals.

Can occasionally cause symptoms of dizziness or lightheadedness, especially if the pauses are prolonged.

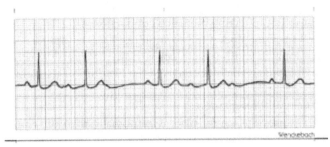

Wenckebach

### History and Discovery
Dr. Karel Frederik Wenckebach: The phenomenon was first described by the Austrian physician Karel Frederik Wenckebach, who initially reported it in 1899. Wenckebach's initial observations were based on the irregular pulse patterns in patients, which he meticulously documented before the widespread use of the ECG.

Dr. Woldemar Mobitz: The classification of AV blocks into Type I and Type II was later refined by Woldemar Mobitz in the 1920s. Mobitz's work, which utilized electrocardiography, provided a clearer understanding of the differences between the two types of second-degree AV block.

## Second-Degree AV Block: Type II (Mobitz II)
### Overview
Type II Second-Degree AV Block, also known as Mobitz II, is a cardiac conduction disorder characterized by the intermittent failure of electrical impulses to conduct from the atria to the ventricles without prior lengthening of the PR interval, which is a key distinguishing factor from Mobitz I.

### ECG Characteristics
Fixed PR Intervals: In Mobitz II, the PR intervals of conducted beats are constant and do not show the progressive prolongation seen in Mobitz I.

Dropped Beats: Some P waves are not followed by QRS complexes, reflecting the failed conduction.

Narrow or Wide QRS Complexes: QRS complexes can be normal in width if the block is at the AV nodal level but may be wide if the blockage is in the His-Purkinje system.

Clinical Presentation

Symptoms: Can be more symptomatic than Mobitz I, with episodes of dizziness, lightheadedness, or syncope due to the sudden and unpredictable nature of the dropped beats.

Risk of Progression: More likely than Mobitz I to progress to complete heart block.

**Pathophysiology**

Site of Block: Unlike Mobitz I, which typically occurs at the AV node, Mobitz II often occurs below the AV node, in the His-Purkinje system.

Failure of Conduction: The underlying mechanism involves the failure of some electrical impulses to conduct through the damaged conduction pathway, despite a normal or near-normal conduction time.

**Management**

Close Monitoring: Given its potential to progress to complete heart block, Mobitz II is often taken more seriously than Mobitz I.

Pacemaker Implantation: Patients with Mobitz II, especially those with symptoms, are often considered for pacemaker implantation as this type of AV block can signify more extensive conduction system disease.

**Clinical Significance**

Indicator of Serious Disease: Mobitz II may indicate more significant heart disease and carries a higher risk of progression to complete heart block than Mobitz I.

Need for Intervention: Due to its potential severity and unpredictability, Mobitz II is more likely to require active intervention, such as pacemaker placement, especially in symptomatic patients or those with structural heart disease.

Mobitz II is considered a more serious form of AV block due to its association with distal conduction system disease and its tendency to progress to more severe forms of heart block. Prompt recognition and appropriate management are crucial to prevent potential complications.

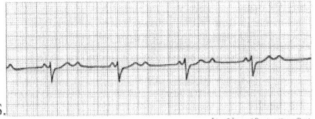

Type II Second Degree Heart Block

### Elaboration on Mobitz I (Wenckebach) and Mobitz II Heart Rate, and their Irregularity/Regularity

**Mobitz I (Wenckebach) Block**

Heart Rate:

Atrial Rate: Typically, within the normal range **(60-100 bpm)**, as the sinus node usually functions normally.

Ventricular Rate: Generally, near normal but can be slightly slower due to dropped beats. The ventricular rate can vary widely depending on the frequency of the Wenckebach cycles (dropped beats).

Regularity:

Atrial Rhythm: Regular, as it follows the normal sinus rhythm.

Ventricular Rhythm: Irregular. The progressive prolongation of the PR interval followed by a non-conducted P wave (dropped beat) leads to an irregular ventricular rhythm.

PR Interval:

The PR interval progressively lengthens with each beat until a beat is dropped. After the dropped beat, the cycle restarts with a shorter PR interval. The specific intervals depend on the individual patient and the severity of the AV nodal delay.

### Mobitz II Block
Heart Rate:

Atrial Rate: Remains normal, typically within the range of **60-100 bpm**.

Ventricular Rate: Often slower than the atrial rate and can be more consistent than in Mobitz I. The rate depends on the ratio of conducted to non-conducted beats (e.g., 2:1, 3:1 block, etc.).

Regularity:

Atrial Rhythm: Regular.

Ventricular Rhythm: Can be regular or irregular. If there is a consistent pattern of conduction and block (like a 2:1 or 3:1 block), the ventricular rhythm may appear regular. However, if the pattern of blocked beats is variable, the ventricular rhythm will be irregular.

PR Interval:

The PR interval in the conducted beats remains constant and does not change as in Wenckebach. The ventricular rate is determined by how many atrial beats are conducted – for example, in a 2:1 block, every second P wave is conducted.

### Key Points
Mobitz I (Wenckebach) is often characterized by a slightly irregular ventricular rhythm due to the cyclical nature of the conduction disturbance, with varying heart rates depending on the frequency of the non-conducted beats.

Mobitz II may have a more regular or predictable ventricular rhythm if there is a consistent pattern of conduction and block but can become irregular if the pattern varies. The ventricular rate in Mobitz II is generally slower than the atrial rate and can vary based on the ratio of conducted to non-conducted atrial impulses.

## Third-Degree (Complete) AV Block

Third-Degree AV Block, also known as Complete Heart Block, is the most severe form of AV block. It occurs when there is a complete disconnection in the electrical conduction between the atria and ventricles.

Characteristics
Complete Dissociation: The atria and ventricles beat independently of each other. The atrial impulses do not conduct to the ventricles.

ECG Findings:
Atrial Rate: Regular with normal P waves, reflecting normal sinus node function.

Ventricular Rate: Also regular, but slower and unrelated to the atrial rate. The ventricles are paced by an escape rhythm originating from the AV junction or ventricles.

Dissociation of P Waves and QRS Complexes: P waves and QRS complexes appear at their own regular but independent rates.

### Heart Rate and Regularity

Atrial Rate: Typically, normal (60-100 beats per minute), as it's controlled by the sinus node.

Ventricular Rate: Varies depending on the site of the escape pacemaker. If the escape rhythm originates from the AV junction, the ventricular rate may be 40-60 beats per minute. If it comes from the ventricles, the rate is usually slower (20-40 beats per minute).

Regularity: Both atrial and ventricular rhythms are regular, but they are not synchronized with each other.

### Clinical Presentation

Symptoms: Can be asymptomatic if the ventricular rate is adequate. However, symptoms often include fatigue, dizziness, lightheadedness, and in severe cases, syncope (fainting) due to reduced cardiac output.

**Severity:** Considered a medical emergency if it leads to hemodynamic instability.

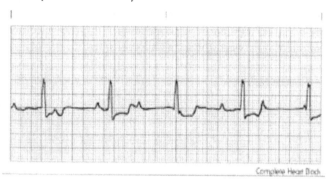

Complete Heart Block

## 2-AV Dissociation and its Implications

### Definition of AV Dissociation

Atrioventricular (AV) Dissociation occurs when the atria and ventricles beat independently of each other. This is not necessarily indicative of a block but rather a lack of coordination in the timing of atrial and ventricular activities.

Characteristics of AV Dissociation

Independence of Atria and Ventricles: The atria are typically paced by the sinus node, while the ventricles may be paced by an ectopic pacemaker or an escape rhythm.

ECG Findings: The ECG shows P waves and QRS complexes that are not related; P waves bear no consistent relationship to the QRS complexes.

## Types:

Interference Dissociation: Occurs when the rate of an ectopic pacemaker in the ventricles is close to or slightly faster than the sinus node rate.

Isorhythmic Dissociation: Happens when the atrial and ventricular rhythms are close in rate and occasionally align, but are not synchronously driven.

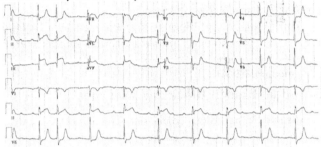

## Comparison with Third-Degree (Complete) AV Block

Third-Degree AV Block

Complete Disconnection: There is a total disconnection in the electrical communication between the atria and ventricles.

ECG Findings: Regular P waves with a rate set by the sinus node and regular QRS complexes with a rate set by a ventricular or junctional escape rhythm, but no relation between the two.

Severity: This is a more serious condition as it often indicates significant conduction system disease and can lead to reduced cardiac output.

### Differences

Origin of Rhythms:

In AV Dissociation, the atrial rhythm is usually normal, and the ventricular rhythm is often an escape rhythm but can be due to other causes like ventricular tachycardia.

In Third-Degree AV Block, the ventricular rhythm is always an escape rhythm due to the failure of atrial impulses to reach the ventricles.

Mechanism:
AV Dissociation can occur without any block in the conduction system. It's more about the timing and rate of atrial and ventricular pacemakers.
Third-Degree AV Block is characterized by a block in the conduction system, preventing atrial impulses from reaching the ventricles.

## 3-Bundle Branch Block and its Types

Bundle Branch Block (BBB) occurs when there is a delay or obstruction along the pathway that electrical impulses travel to make your heart beat. The heart has two main branches in its electrical conduction system - the right and left bundle branches. When one of these branches is blocked, it causes a delay in the electrical conduction to the respective ventricle.

### Right Bundle Branch Block (RBBB)
### Characteristics:
ECG Findings: A hallmark of RBBB is the presence of a wide QRS complex (>0.12 seconds). In lead V1, there is typically an 'R' wave or a 'bunny ear' appearance. In lead V6, a wide, slurred S wave is observed.
Conduction: The right ventricle is activated later than the left ventricle.
Implications: RBBB can be a normal variant in healthy individuals, especially in the absence of other cardiac abnormalities. However, it can also be associated with conditions like right ventricular hypertrophy, pulmonary embolism, or ischemic heart disease.

### Left Bundle Branch Block (LBBB)
### Characteristics:

ECG Findings: In LBBB, there is also a widening of the QRS complex (>0.12 seconds). In leads V1 and V2, broad, deep S waves are present. In leads I, aVL, V5, and V6, there are typically tall, broad 'R' waves.

Conduction: The left ventricle is activated later than the right ventricle.

Implications: LBBB is more likely to indicate heart disease, particularly in older adults. It is often associated with conditions like left ventricular hypertrophy, hypertension, aortic valve disease, or cardiomyopathies.

## Clinical Significance

Symptoms: Bundle branch blocks themselves may not cause any symptoms. However, they can be indicative of underlying heart disease, which may present with symptoms like shortness of breath, fatigue, or chest pain.

Diagnosis: Diagnosed through an ECG. The specific pattern of the QRS complex widening helps in distinguishing between RBBB and LBBB.

Management: Management of BBB focuses primarily on treating any underlying heart conditions. The presence of a bundle branch block can impact the interpretation of ECGs, especially in diagnosing myocardial infarctions.

## Key Considerations

Progression to More Severe Blocks: In some cases, a bundle branch block may progress to more severe forms of heart block or can complicate other arrhythmias.

Importance in Clinical Settings: Recognition of BBB is crucial in clinical settings as it can influence decisions regarding the use of certain medications and the need for pacemaker implantation.

In summary, bundle branch blocks are significant findings on an ECG that can be either benign or indicative of various cardiac pathologies. The type of BBB (whether right or left) provides clues to the underlying cardiac condition and helps guide further evaluation and management.

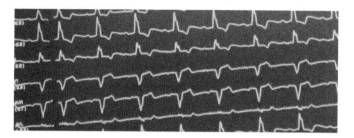

## 4- Blocked Premature Atrial Contractions (Blocked PACs)

Definition

Blocked Premature Atrial Contractions (PACs) are early electrical impulses originating from the atria that do not conduct through to the ventricles. In other words, these are premature beats from the atria that fail to result in a subsequent ventricular contraction.

Characteristics

ECG Findings:

Presence of an Early P Wave: An abnormal P wave, indicating the premature atrial contraction, is visible on the ECG.

Absence of QRS Complex Following the P Wave: Unlike typical PACs where each premature P wave is followed by a QRS complex, in blocked PACs, the QRS complex is absent after the premature P wave.

P-P Interval Disruption: The occurrence of the blocked PAC disrupts the regularity of the atrial rhythm, though the underlying sinus rhythm is usually maintained.

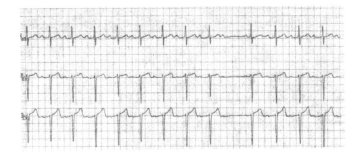

# XI-VENTRICULAR RHYTHMS

1.  Idioventricular Rhythms
2.  Accelerated Idioventricular Rhythm
3.  Ventricular Tachycardia (V-Tach)
4.  Ventricular Fibrillation and Torsade de pointes
5.  Interpolated Premature Ventricular Contractions (PVCs)
6.  Wide Complex Beats and PVCs
7.  Idioventricular Conduction Delay (IVCD) and Aberrancy
8.  . Differences Between Bundle Branch Block (BBB), Idioventricular Conduction Delay (IVCD), and Aberrancy

## 1-Idioventricular Rhythm

Definition

Idioventricular rhythm is a type of cardiac rhythm that originates from the ventricles (the lower chambers of the heart). It is considered a type of escape rhythm that occurs when the sinoatrial (SA) node and atrioventricular (AV) node fail to generate or transmit an impulse, prompting the ventricles to initiate their own rhythm.

Characteristics

Rate: Typically slow, ranging from 20 to 40 beats per minute, though it can sometimes be faster, particularly in accelerated idioventricular rhythm (AIVR), where the rate is between 40 and 100 beats per minute.

ECG Findings:

Wide QRS Complexes: The QRS complexes are wide (>0.12 seconds) and have an abnormal morphology, as the ventricular depolarization does not follow the normal conduction pathway.

Regular Rhythm: The rhythm is usually regular, but the rate is slower than normal sinus rhythm.

Absent P Waves: P waves are typically absent, or if present, are not associated with the QRS complexes, indicating dissociation from atrial activity.

Clinical Implications

Symptoms: Due to the slow rate, patients may experience symptoms of reduced cardiac output, such as dizziness, fatigue, or syncope.

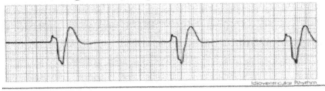

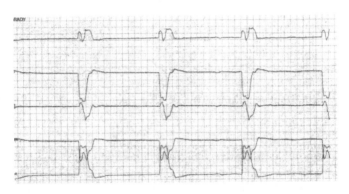

## 2-Accelerated Idioventricular Rhythm (AIVR)

Accelerated Idioventricular Rhythm is a specific type of ventricular rhythm that is faster than the typical idioventricular rhythm but not as fast as ventricular tachycardia. It often occurs transiently and is particularly associated with specific cardiac events and conditions.

Characteristics

Heart Rate: AIVR is characterized by a heart rate that is faster than a typical idioventricular rhythm but slower than ventricular tachycardia, typically ranging from 40 to 100 beats per minute.

ECG Findings:
Wide QRS Complexes: Similar to other ventricular rhythms, the QRS complexes in AIVR are wide (>0.12 seconds) and have an abnormal morphology.

Regular Rhythm: The rhythm tends to be regular, with a consistent rate that is faster than normal ventricular escape rhythms but not reaching the threshold of tachycardia.

P Wave Relationship: P waves may be present but are not associated with the QRS complexes, indicating dissociation from atrial activity

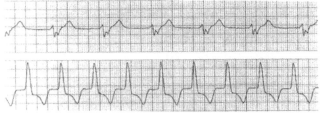

## 3-Ventricular Tachycardia (VT)

Definition
Ventricular Tachycardia is defined as a sequence of three or more consecutive heartbeats originating from the ventricles at a rate exceeding 100 beats per minute. It is a potentially life-threatening arrhythmia due to its impact on cardiac output and its propensity to deteriorate into more serious conditions like ventricular fibrillation.

Characteristics
Heart Rate: The rate in VT typically ranges from 100 to 250 beats per minute, though it can occasionally be higher.

ECG Findings:

Wide QRS Complexes: The QRS complexes in VT are usually wide (>0.12 seconds) and have an abnormal shape.

Regular or Irregular Rhythm: VT can present as a regular or irregular rhythm. Monomorphic VT (where all QRS complexes look similar) typically has a regular rhythm, while polymorphic VT (varying QRS morphology) may be irregular.

**Types of VT**

Monomorphic VT: Characterized by QRS complexes that are similar in shape. It's often associated with structural heart disease like previous myocardial infarction or cardiomyopathy.

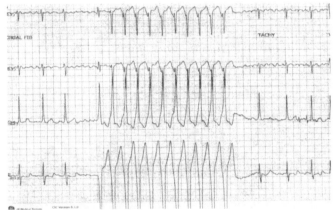

Polymorphic VT: The QRS complexes vary in shape from beat to beat. This form can occur in the context of a prolonged QT interval or other metabolic disturbances.

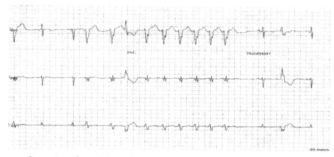

Sustained vs Non-Sustained VT: Sustained VT lasts for more than 30 seconds or requires termination due to hemodynamic instability.

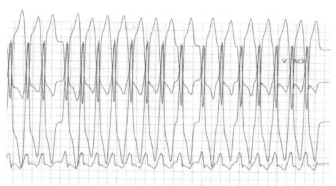

Non-sustained VT lasts less than 30 seconds and stops spontaneously.

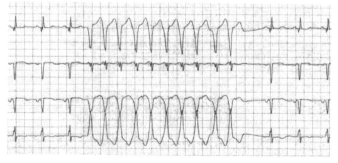

## 4-Ventricular Fibrillation (V-Fib) and Torsade de pointes

Definition

Ventricular Fibrillation (V-Fib) is a life-threatening cardiac arrhythmia characterized by the rapid, irregular, and chaotic electrical activity of the ventricles. This erratic activity results in the loss of coordinated ventricular contractions, leading to a severe decrease in cardiac output and the cessation of effective blood circulation.

ECG Characteristics

Irregular and Chaotic Pattern: The ECG in V-Fib shows a completely irregular and chaotic waveform without any discernible P waves, QRS complexes, or T waves.

Varying Waveform Amplitude: The amplitude of the fibrillatory waves can vary, sometimes described as "coarse" or "fine" V-Fib based on the size of the oscillations.

Mechanism

Disorganized Electrical Activity: In V-Fib, multiple areas of the ventricles simultaneously generate disorganized electrical impulses. This results in the ventricles quivering rather than contracting effectively.

Lack of Effective Contraction: The chaotic electrical activity prevents the heart from pumping blood, leading to immediate hemodynamic collapse.

Clinical Presentation

Sudden Cardiac Arrest: V-Fib typically presents as sudden cardiac arrest, with the patient losing consciousness within seconds. There are no effective heartbeats, no palpable pulse, and no normal blood pressure.

Medical Emergency: V-Fib is a medical emergency that requires immediate intervention, as it can lead to death within minutes if not promptly treated.

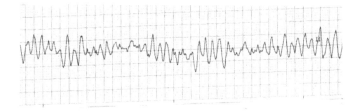

## Torsade de Pointes
Definition

Torsade de Pointes, which translates to "twisting of the points," is a specific type of polymorphic ventricular tachycardia. It is characterized by a rapid heart rate and a distinct ECG appearance where the QRS complexes seem to "twist" around the baseline.

### ECG Characteristics
Varying Amplitude: The hallmark of Torsade de Pointes is the variation in the amplitude and polarity of the QRS complexes, which appear to spiral or twist around the ECG baseline.

Heart Rate: Typically, very rapid, often between 200 and 250 beats per minute.

Association with Prolonged QT Interval: It frequently occurs in the context of a prolonged QT interval, which can be congenital or acquired.

### History and Discovery
First Description: Torsade de Pointes was first described by the French cardiologist, François Dessertenne, in 1966. He observed the peculiar ECG pattern in a patient with a prolonged QT interval.

Term Coinage: Dessertenne coined the term "Torsade de Pointes" to describe the characteristic twisting pattern seen on the ECG.

### Mechanism

Triggered Activity: Torsade de Pointes is thought to result from a phenomenon called "triggered activity," which occurs when afterdepolarizations (abnormal depolarizations following the main heart muscle contraction) in the setting of a prolonged QT interval lead to the initiation of abnormal heartbeats.

Role of Prolonged QT Interval: The prolonged QT interval creates an electrophysiological environment conducive to the development of reentrant arrhythmias, which underlie Torsade de Pointes.

### Clinical Implications

Symptoms: Can range from dizziness and palpitations to severe cases of syncope or cardiac arrest.

Risk Factors: Conditions that prolong the QT interval, including certain medications, electrolyte imbalances (like hypokalemia and hypomagnesemia), congenital long QT syndrome, and heart disease.

## 5-Interpolated Premature Ventricular Contractions (PVCs)

Definition

An Interpolated PVC is a type of premature ventricular contraction that occurs early in the cardiac cycle but does not disrupt the normal sinus rhythm. It is "interpolated" between two regular heartbeats without causing a

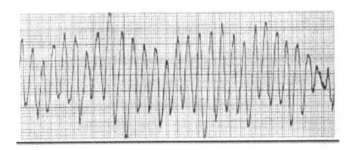

compensatory pause, which is typically seen with other types of PVCs.

ECG Characteristics

Early Wide QRS Complex: On the ECG, an interpolated PVC is identified by an early, wide, and aberrant QRS complex, characteristic of ventricular origin.

No Compensatory Pause: Unlike typical PVCs, interpolated PVCs are followed immediately by a normal sinus beat, resulting in no compensatory pause.

Normal Sinus Beats Before and After: The PVC is sandwiched between two normal sinus beats, and the sinus rhythm is maintained before and after the PVC.

Mechanism

Timing: The timing of the PVC is such that it falls early enough in the cardiac cycle so that the ventricles have time to repolarize before the arrival of the next sinus impulse.

Ventricular Excitation: The ventricles are prematurely excited by the PVC, but the sinus node continues its normal pacing, unaware of the ventricular activity.

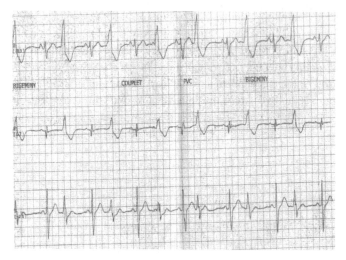

## 6-Wide Complex Tachycardia

Definition
Wide Complex Tachycardia (WCT) refers to any tachycardia (rapid heart rate) with a broad QRS complex (greater than 0.12 seconds) on an electrocardiogram (ECG). WCT is a categorization based on ECG findings and includes several potential arrhythmias, with Ventricular Tachycardia (VT) being the most common and significant.

Characteristics
Heart Rate: Generally, over 100 beats per minute.
QRS Duration: More than 0.12 seconds, indicating a ventricular origin or abnormal conduction.
Rhythm: Can be regular or irregular.

### Types of Wide Complex Tachycardia

Ventricular Tachycardia (VT): As discussed previously, originates from the ventricles and is the most common form of WCT.

Supraventricular Tachycardia (SVT) with Aberrancy: This includes atrial fibrillation, atrial flutter, and other SVTs with abnormal conduction through the ventricles.

Pre-excited Tachycardias: Such as those seen in Wolff-Parkinson-White (WPW) syndrome where an accessory pathway bypasses the normal AV nodal conduction.

Pacemaker-Induced Tachycardia: In patients with pacemakers, certain pacing modes can produce wide QRS complexes.

### Comparison with Ventricular Tachycardia (VT)

VT as a Subset of WCT: VT is a specific diagnosis within the broader category of WCT. Not all WCTs are VTs, but VT is the most critical diagnosis to consider when a WCT is identified.

Origin and Mechanism: VT originates from the ventricles, often due to underlying heart disease or scar tissue. Other WCTs may originate above the ventricles but display a wide QRS due to aberrant conduction.

# 7-Idioventricular Conduction Delay and Aberrancy

Definition

Idioventricular Conduction Delay refers to a delay in the conduction of electrical impulses within the ventricles. This delay is not due to a block at the level of the AV node but occurs within the ventricular conduction system itself.

Characteristics

ECG Findings: Typically characterized by a widened QRS complex (>0.12 seconds) indicating delayed ventricular depolarization.

Underlying Causes: Often associated with structural abnormalities in the ventricles, such as scar tissue from a previous myocardial infarction, cardiomyopathies, or congenital abnormalities in the conduction system.

Clinical Implications: While it may not produce symptoms on its own, idioventricular conduction delay can be an important marker of underlying heart disease and may affect the heart's efficiency in pumping blood.

## Aberrant Conduction (Aberrancy)

Definition

Aberrant Conduction, often referred to as "Aberrancy," occurs when the electrical impulses in the heart follow an unusual pathway or timing, leading to a change in the QRS complex's shape and duration.

Characteristics

ECG Findings: Aberrancy often manifests as a widened QRS complex, similar to a bundle branch block pattern. However, unlike a true bundle branch block, aberrancy can be intermittent and depends on the heart rate or rhythm.

**Types:**

Rate-Related Aberrancy: Often seen in conditions like supraventricular tachycardia (SVT), where the rapid heart rate leads to transient abnormal ventricular conduction.

Ashman Phenomenon: A specific type of aberrancy seen in atrial fibrillation, where a sudden change in the R-R interval leads to a wide QRS complex.

### Clinical Implications

Misdiagnosis Concerns: Aberrant conduction can mimic ventricular tachycardia on an ECG, leading to potential misdiagnosis.

Underlying Causes: Aberrancy can be seen in healthy individuals but is more common in the presence of underlying heart disease, electrolyte imbalances, or drug effects.

Comparison and Implications

Similarity in ECG Presentation: Both idioventricular conduction delay and aberrancy can present with widened QRS complexes, but the underlying mechanisms are different.

Idioventricular Conduction Delay: Indicates a more fixed and localized issue within the ventricles' conduction system.

Aberrant Conduction: More often related to the rate or rhythm of the heart and can be more variable

## 8- Differences Between Bundle Branch Block (BBB), Idioventricular Conduction Delay (IVCD), and Aberrancy

Understanding the differences between Bundle Branch Block (BBB), Idioventricular Conduction Delay (IVCD), and Aberrant Conduction (Aberrancy) is crucial in cardiology, as each has distinct implications for cardiac function and health.

## Bundle Branch Block (BBB)

Definition: A BBB occurs when there is a delay or blockage in the electrical conduction through either the right or left bundle branches, which are the main pathways for electrical flow to the left and right ventricles.

ECG Characteristics:

Right BBB (RBBB): Characterized by a wide QRS complex (>0.12 seconds), with a distinctive 'R' wave or 'rabbit ears' in V1 and a wide, slurred S wave in lead I and V6.

Left BBB (LBBB): Also shows a wide QRS complex, with a broad, monophasic 'R' wave in leads I, aVL, V5, and V6, and deep S waves in V1.

Clinical Implications: Can be associated with underlying heart disease, particularly LBBB. It affects the synchronization of ventricular contraction.

## Idioventricular Conduction Delay (IVCD)

Definition: IVCD refers to a delay in the conduction within the ventricles, which is not localized to the bundle branches. It's a more diffuse or generalized impairment of ventricular conduction.

ECG Characteristics: Shows a wide QRS complex similar to BBB, but without the typical patterns associated with either RBBB or LBBB.

Clinical Significance: Indicates a global ventricular conduction impairment and can be associated with various cardiac pathologies, including cardiomyopathies and diffuse myocardial damage.

## Aberrant Conduction (Aberrancy)

Definition: Aberrant conduction refers to a situation where the electrical impulse follows an unusual pathway or timing through the ventricles, leading to a temporary alteration in the QRS complex's shape and duration.

ECG Characteristics: Presents as a wide QRS complex that may mimic BBB, often occurring intermittently and dependent on heart rate or rhythm (e.g., Ashman phenomenon in atrial fibrillation).

Clinical Implications: Often a transient phenomenon and can be seen in healthy individuals, though it may also occur in the context of underlying heart disease. It's particularly important in the differential diagnosis of ventricular tachycardia.

Key Differences
Localization:
BBB: Localized to the right or left bundle branches.
IVCD: More diffuse delay within the ventricles, not confined to the bundle branches.
Aberrancy: A temporary and rate-dependent conduction abnormality, not a fixed block.

ECG Patterns:
BBB: Specific ECG patterns are associated with RBBB and LBBB.
IVCD: Wide QRS without the specific patterns of RBBB or LBBB.
Aberrancy: Wide QRS that can vary and often appears intermittently.

Clinical Context:
BBB: Often indicates underlying structural heart disease.
IVCD: Suggests more generalized ventricular conduction impairment.
Aberrancy: Can be a benign, transient phenomenon but requires careful assessment to rule out more serious conditions.

Differentiating these conditions on an ECG is crucial for appropriate clinical management and understanding the patient's underlying cardiac health. Each present with a wide

QRS complex, but the patterns, consistency, and associated clinical contexts help in distinguishing them.

# XII-PACEMAKER RHYTHMS

1.    Pacemaker overview
2.    Types of Pacemaker Rhythms: A-Paced, V-Paced, AV-Paced, Bi-Ventricular Paced
3.    Failure to pace
4.    Failure to Sense, Under/Oversensing, Overdrive Pacing
5.    Pacemaker-Mediated Tachycardia, Cross Talk
6.    Wandering Atrial Pacemaker

## 1-Pacemaker: Overview

A pacemaker is a small medical device that's implanted in the chest to help manage irregular heartbeats, known as arrhythmias. It's primarily used in conditions where the heart beats too slowly (bradycardia), too fast (tachycardia), or irregularly.

How It Works
Electrical Impulses: A pacemaker sends electrical impulses to the heart to ensure it beats at a regular rate and rhythm.

Sensing Heartbeats: Modern pacemakers can also "sense" the heart's natural electrical activity and only deliver impulses when necessary.

### Types of Pacemakers
Single-Chamber Pacemakers: Stimulate either the right atrium or the right ventricle.

Dual-Chamber Pacemakers: Stimulate both the right atrium and right ventricle, allowing coordination between the chambers.

Biventricular Pacemakers (Cardiac Resynchronization Therapy): Used in heart failure, stimulating both ventricles to improve the efficiency of the heart's contractions.

### Indications for Use

Bradycardia: When the heart beats too slowly.

Heart Block: A condition where the electrical signal is delayed or blocked after leaving the SA node.

Atrial Fibrillation: To regulate the heart rate, particularly when medications are ineffective.

Heart Failure: To improve heart function and symptoms.

### Components

Pulse Generator: Contains the battery and the circuitry that controls the rate of electrical pulse generation.

Leads: Wires that deliver the electrical pulses to the heart. They also relay information about the heart's natural activity back to the device.

### Implantation Procedure

A pacemaker implantation is typically a minimally invasive surgery, often performed under local anesthesia.

Leads are inserted into a vein and guided to the heart, and the pulse generator is placed under the skin in the chest.

### Living with a Pacemaker

Regular Monitoring: Pacemakers require regular check-ups to ensure they are functioning correctly and to monitor the battery life.

Lifestyle Considerations: Most individuals with pacemakers can lead normal lives, though they may need to avoid certain electrical devices or strong magnetic fields.

### Risks and Complications

Risks include infection, bleeding, and, rarely, damage to the heart or blood vessels.

There can be issues with the device, such as malfunctions or battery depletion.

## Technological Advances

Modern pacemakers have advanced features like rate responsiveness, adjusting the pacing rate based on physical activity.

Remote monitoring capabilities allow for data transmission to healthcare providers from a patient's home.

## Summary

Pacemakers play a vital role in managing certain heart rhythm disorders, significantly improving the quality of life for many patients with cardiac arrhythmias. With advancements in technology, pacemakers have become more efficient, reliable, and compatible with a patient's daily activities. Regular medical follow-up is essential for optimal management of a pacemaker.

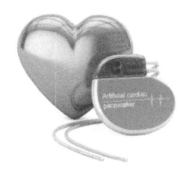

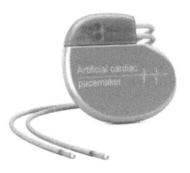

## 2-Types of Pacemaker Rhythms

### Single Chamber Pacing:

**Atrial Pacing:** Characterized by a pacing spike followed by a P wave. The QRS complex usually follows normally.

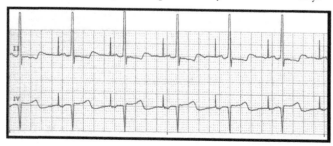

**Ventricular Pacing**: Exhibits a pacing spike followed by a wide QRS complex. No association with the P wave, as the atria are not paced.

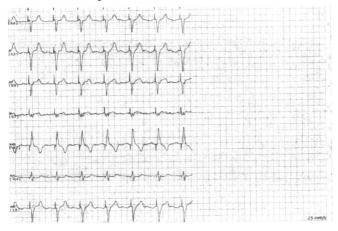

## Dual Chamber Pacing:

Sequential Pacing: Pacing spikes precede both the P wave and the QRS complex, indicating pacing of both atria and ventricles.

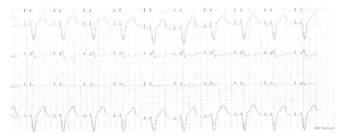

Synchronized Pacing: Coordinates atrial and ventricular contractions to maintain an optimal atrioventricular delay.

**Biventricular Pacing:**

Used in Cardiac Resynchronization Therapy (CRT) for heart failure.

Pacing spikes precede synchronized contractions of both ventricles to improve cardiac efficiency.

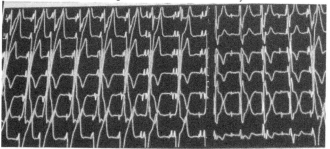

# 3-Failure to Pace (Non-Pacing) and Failure to Capture

Definition

Failure to Pace, also known as Non-Pacing, occurs when a pacemaker does not deliver an electrical impulse when it is supposed to. This malfunction can lead to a lack of adequate cardiac pacing, which may result in a slower than desired heart rate or pauses in the heart rhythm.

ECG Characteristics

**Absence of Pacing Spikes**: On the ECG, this condition is identified by the lack of expected pacing spikes.

Resulting Heart Rhythm: The patient's underlying heart rhythm will be apparent, which may be abnormally slow or irregular if the patient is dependent on the pacemaker.

Causes

Battery Depletion: The most common cause is the end of the battery life, where the pacemaker no longer has the power to generate pacing impulses.

Lead Issues: Dislodgement, fracture, or disconnection of the pacemaker leads can prevent electrical impulses from being delivered to the heart muscle.

Circuit Malfunction: Internal malfunction of the pacemaker's circuitry can inhibit its ability to pace.

Programming Error: Incorrect programming of the pacemaker can result in failure to deliver appropriate pacing impulses.

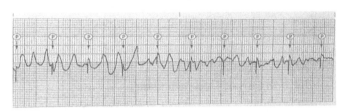

### Failure to Capture:

Description: The pacemaker delivers a pacing impulse, but the heart muscle does not respond.

ECG Findings: Pacing spikes without a subsequent P wave or QRS complex.

Causes: Lead dislodgement, high pacing threshold, or lead fracture.

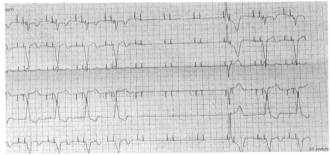

# 4-Failure to Sense (Under-Sensing or Over-Sensing):

### Under-Sensing in Pacemakers
Definition

Under-sensing is a malfunction in pacemaker behavior where the device fails to detect (sense) the heart's natural electrical activity. When a pacemaker under-senses, it does not recognize spontaneous cardiac events (like intrinsic heartbeats), potentially leading to inappropriate pacing.

## How Pacemakers Should Normally Function

Sensing: A properly functioning pacemaker continuously monitors the heart's intrinsic electrical activity.

Pacing Decisions: Based on this sensing, the pacemaker decides whether to deliver an electrical impulse to stimulate a heartbeat.

## The Problem of Under-Sensing

Inappropriate Pacing: When under-sensing occurs, the pacemaker may falsely assume that the heart's intrinsic rate is too slow or absent, leading to unnecessary pacing.

Risk: This can result in pacing during the heart's natural contraction cycle, potentially causing arrhythmias or inefficient heart function.

## ECG Characteristics of Under-Sensing

Pacing Spikes in Presence of Intrinsic Rhythm: On an ECG, you might see pacing spikes occurring even though there are normal heartbeats present. The pacemaker is essentially 'ignoring' the heart's own electrical activity.

Potential Overlap with T-Wave: A pacing stimulus could fall on the T-wave of the intrinsic heartbeat, potentially leading to a dangerous arrhythmia called "R-on-T" phenomenon.

## Causes of Under-Sensing

Lead Issues: Displacement, fracture, or malfunction of the pacing lead can impair sensing.

Device Programming: Inappropriate sensitivity settings in the pacemaker programming.

Electrode Issues: Problems with the electrode-tissue interface, such as fibrosis at the electrode site.

Battery Depletion: Sometimes, low battery power can affect the pacemaker's ability to sense properly.

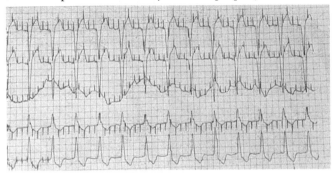

## Over-Sensing in Pacemakers

Definition

Over-sensing in pacemakers refers to a condition where the pacemaker mistakenly detects electrical signals that are not true cardiac activity (non-cardiac electrical activity) and, as a result, inappropriately inhibits its pacing function.

How It Occurs

**Extraneous Electrical Signals:** The pacemaker can pick up electrical signals from sources other than the heart. These can include muscular activity (myopotentials), external electromagnetic interference, or even internal pacemaker component malfunction.

**Sensitivity Setting:** Over-sensing is often related to the sensitivity setting of the pacemaker. If the device is set too sensitive, it may detect small electrical signals that it should normally ignore.

## ECG Characteristics

Inappropriate Pauses: The ECG may show pauses where the pacemaker fails to pace because it incorrectly senses electrical activity.

Inconsistent Pacing: The pacing may appear erratic, not aligning with the programmed pacing intervals due to the pacemaker intermittently inhibiting its output.

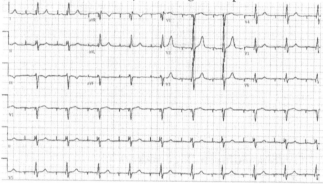

## Overdrive Pacing

Definition

Overdrive pacing is a cardiac pacing technique where the heart is stimulated to beat at a rate faster than its intrinsic rhythm. This technique is primarily used in the management of certain arrhythmias.

Mechanism

- **Increased Pacing Rate**: A pacemaker or an external pacing device delivers electrical impulses at a rate higher than the heart's natural rhythm.

- **Suppression of Arrhythmias**: The rapid pacing effectively overrides abnormal rhythms, especially those originating from ectopic foci (areas outside the normal conduction pathway).

Clinical Applications

1. **Tachyarrhythmias**: Particularly effective in treating tachyarrhythmias that originate from

automatic foci, including certain types of atrial and ventricular tachycardias.

2. **Atrial Fibrillation**: Sometimes used to convert atrial fibrillation to a normal sinus rhythm, especially when other treatments are ineffective.

3. **Re-entrant Arrhythmias**: Can interrupt re-entrant circuits, a common cause of tachyarrhythmias.

Procedure

- **Temporary or Permanent Pacemaker:** Overdrive pacing can be administered through an external pacemaker or a permanently implanted device.

- **Rate Adjustment:** The pacing rate is set higher than the patient's intrinsic heart rate but within a safe range to prevent adverse effects.

## 5-Pacemaker-Mediated Tachycardia and Cross-Talk

Description: A pacemaker-induced arrhythmia, often due to inappropriate sensing or pacing.

ECG Findings: Rapid pacing rate, potentially leading to tachycardia.

Overshooting or Runaway Pacemaker:

Description: Rare malfunction where the pacemaker generates a pacing rate much higher than programmed.

ECG Findings: Very rapid pacing spikes.

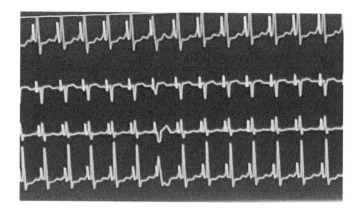

**Cross-Talk:**

In Dual-Chamber Systems: Occurs when an atrial pacing spike is inappropriately sensed by the ventricular lead, inhibiting ventricular pacing.

ECG Findings: Atrial pacing without subsequent ventricular pacing.

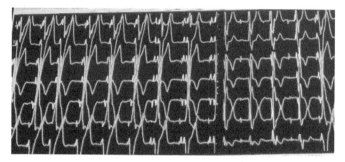

Management of Pacemaker Malfunctions

Diagnosis: Regular pacemaker checks, interrogation, and ECG monitoring are essential to diagnose and manage malfunctions.

Intervention: May include reprogramming the pacemaker, adjusting sensitivity settings, or in some cases, surgical intervention for lead or battery issues.

Preventive Measures: Regular follow-up, avoiding close proximity to strong electromagnetic fields, and awareness of symptoms that may indicate malfunction.

## Summary
Understanding pacemaker rhythms and the various types of malfunctions is essential for ensuring the device functions properly and provides the intended cardiac support. Regular monitoring and maintenance are crucial, as is prompt attention to any signs of malfunction.

# Oversensing and Undersensing in Pacemakers
Pacemakers are designed to maintain regular cardiac rhythm by delivering electrical impulses to the heart. Two common issues that can arise with pacemaker function are oversensing and undersensing, both involving the device's ability to accurately detect the heart's intrinsic electrical activity.

## Oversensing
Definition: Oversensing occurs when the pacemaker detects electrical signals that are not true heartbeats (extracardiac signals) and erroneously interprets these as intrinsic cardiac activities.

Mechanism: The pacemaker becomes too sensitive and picks up on electrical noise or myopotentials (muscle activity), mistaking them for heartbeats.

ECG Characteristics: Inappropriate pauses in pacing where the pacemaker inhibits its output due to the false detection of cardiac activity.

Implications: Can lead to inappropriate inhibition of pacing, resulting in periods of bradycardia (slow heart rate) or asystole (absence of heartbeats), especially if the patient is dependent on the pacemaker.

Management: Adjusting the sensitivity settings of the pacemaker and ensuring proper lead placement.

### Undersensing

Definition: Undersensing occurs when the pacemaker fails to detect the heart's intrinsic electrical activity.

Mechanism: The pacemaker's sensitivity is too low, causing it to miss the heart's natural electrical signals.

ECG Characteristics: The pacemaker continues to pace the heart regardless of the intrinsic rhythm, which can lead to pacing spikes occurring on top of the heart's natural QRS complexes (R-on-T phenomenon) or other inappropriate times.

Implications: May lead to a risk of arrhythmias, including potentially dangerous ones like ventricular tachycardia, especially if the pacemaker triggers a beat on a vulnerable part of the cardiac cycle.

Management: Involves reprogramming the pacemaker to correctly sense the heart's intrinsic electrical activity and potentially adjusting lead placement.

### Key Differences
### Nature of Sensing Issue:

Oversensing: The pacemaker is too sensitive, detecting extraneous signals as heartbeats.

Undersensing: The pacemaker is not sensitive enough, failing to detect actual heartbeats.

### Resulting Pacemaker Behavior:

Oversensing: Inappropriate inhibition of pacemaker output, leading to pauses in pacing.

Undersensing: Inappropriate pacing without regard for the heart's natural rhythm, potentially pacing during the heart's vulnerable period.

## 6-Wandering Atrial Pacemaker

Definition

A Wandering Atrial Pacemaker (WAP) is a cardiac rhythm where the pacemaking impulse shifts between the sinoatrial (SA) node, the atria, and the atrioventricular (AV) junction. This shift in pacemaker sites results in a rhythm that is generally normal in rate but variable in rhythm due to the changing origin of **the electrical impulse.**

### ECG Characteristics
Variable P Wave Morphology: The most distinguishing feature is the variability in P wave shape and size, reflecting the changing site of atrial activation.

Irregular Atrial Rate: The atrial rhythm can be irregular, with a varying P-P interval.

Normal or Slightly Irregular Ventricular Rate: The ventricular rate is usually normal, though it can be slightly irregular due to the irregular atrial pacing.

Normal or Variable PR Interval: Depending on the origin of the impulse, the PR interval can change; impulses originating closer to the AV node will have a shorter PR interval.

### Clinical Context
Common in Healthy Individuals: WAP is often seen in healthy people, especially the young and the elderly, and is generally considered a benign variant.

Association with Respiratory Patterns: It can be associated with respiratory patterns, often more pronounced during deep breathing, a phenomenon known as respiratory sinus arrhythmia.

### Clinical Implications
Symptoms: Typically, asymptomatic, WAP usually does not cause any noticeable symptoms.

Significance: It is not associated with any significant cardiac pathology and does not usually require treatment.

Management

Observation: WAP generally only requires observation. No specific treatment is necessary in most cases.

Lifestyle Modifications: In some instances, lifestyle modifications to improve overall cardiovascular health might be recommended.

Regular Monitoring: If there are any concerns or if the patient has other cardiac conditions, regular monitoring may be advised.

### Differentiation from Other Arrhythmias

Distinguishing from Atrial Fibrillation or Flutter: It is important to differentiate WAP from other atrial arrhythmias like atrial fibrillation or flutter, which have different implications and require different management strategies.

**Absence of Rapid Rate:** Unlike atrial tachycardia or atrial flutter, WAP does not present with a rapid heart rate.

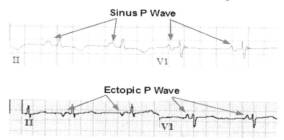

Summary

A wandering Atrial Pacemaker is a rhythm characterized by a shift in the pacemaking impulse among various sites within the atria. It is generally benign and asymptomatic, often requiring no treatment other than observation. Recognizing WAP is important for distinguishing it from more serious atrial arrhythmias.

# XIII. CARDIAC ARREST RHYTHMS

1. Pause, Standstill, and Asystole
2. Agonal Rhythm and its Implications

## 1-Pause, Standstill, and Asystole

### Pause

Definition: A pause in cardiac rhythm is a temporary cessation of cardiac electrical activity. It's a gap in the normal rhythm sequence where a beat is expected but does not occur.

ECG Characteristics: An absence of both P waves and QRS complexes for a duration that is longer than a normal beat interval but typically not exceeding a few seconds.

Duration:
The specific duration that constitutes a pause can vary, but it's often defined as a missing beat or a gap in the rhythm that is at least twice the normal P-P or R-R interval.

A common benchmark is a gap of 2-3 seconds or more.

Clinical Significance:
Short pauses (a few seconds) can be seen in healthy individuals, particularly during sleep.

Longer pauses may indicate an underlying heart condition and can lead to symptoms like dizziness or syncope.

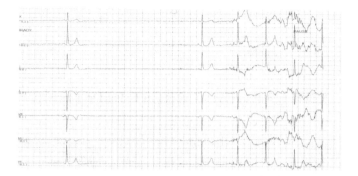

## Standstill

Definition: Cardiac standstill is an extended period of no cardiac electrical activity.

ECG Characteristics: A prolonged flatline on the ECG with no discernible electrical activity.

Duration:

When the duration of a pause extends beyond just a few seconds and approaches or exceeds 20-30 seconds, it is often considered a standstill.

Clinical Significance:

This is a critical condition and essentially represents a form of cardiac arrest.

Immediate medical intervention is necessary.

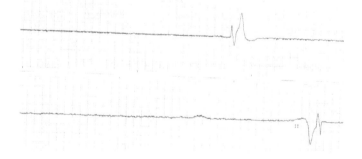

## Asystole

Definition: Asystole is the complete absence of any cardiac electrical activity, often referred to as a "flatline."

ECG Characteristics:

Characterized by a straight line on an ECG, indicating no electrical activity in the heart.

Clinical Significance:

Asystole is a terminal rhythm, typically seen in the final stages of cardiac arrest.

Resuscitation efforts, including CPR and administration of medications like epinephrine, are indicated, but the prognosis is generally poor.

## Key Points
### Pause vs. Standstill vs. Asystole:

Pause: A temporary and relatively short cessation of cardiac rhythm, usually lasting a few seconds.

Standstill: An extended cessation of cardiac rhythm, approaching or exceeding 20-30 seconds, and is a more severe form of cardiac arrest.

Asystole: The most severe and sustained absence of cardiac electrical activity, typically irreversible and associated with terminal stages of cardiac arrest.

Management and Implications:

Short pauses might require no intervention or could indicate a need for pacing in the context of recurring or symptomatic events.

Cardiac standstill and asystole require immediate emergency medical intervention, though the success of resuscitation in asystole is limited.

## 2-Agonal Rhythm

Definition
Agonal rhythm refers to a sporadic, irregular cardiac rhythm often seen in the context of severe hypoxia or cardiac arrest. It represents a state of minimal and ineffective cardiac activity, typically observed in the dying heart.

### ECG Characteristics

Irregular, Widened QRS Complexes: The QRS complexes are irregular, often widened, and appear at a markedly slow rate.

**Rhythm Pattern:** The pattern is erratic, with no consistent P waves or regular rhythm. The rate is usually very slow, often less than 20 beats per minute.

Low Amplitude: The electrical activity is generally of low amplitude, reflecting the heart's depleted energy state.

Clinical Context
End-Stage Cardiac Arrest: Agonal rhythm is usually seen in end-stage cardiac arrest situations. It is a pre-terminal rhythm, often preceding asystole or complete electrical inactivity.

Severe Hypoxia: The rhythm can also occur in states of severe hypoxia, where the oxygen supply to the heart muscle is critically low.

### Clinical Implications

Prognosis: The presence of an agonal rhythm is a grave sign, typically indicating that cardiac arrest is imminent or already occurring.

Urgency of Treatment: Immediate resuscitative efforts are necessary, including cardiopulmonary resuscitation (CPR) and advanced cardiac life support (ACLS). However, the chances of successful resuscitation are often low, especially if the agonal rhythm has been present for an extended period.

## Management

Cardiopulmonary Resuscitation (CPR): Immediate CPR is crucial to provide circulatory support and oxygenation.

**Advanced Life Support:** Involves the use of medications, airway management, and potentially defibrillation, though agonal rhythm itself is not a shockable rhythm.

Rapid Assessment and Intervention: Quick assessment to identify reversible causes and immediate intervention is critical.

Summary

Agonal rhythm is a critical finding, often indicating imminent cardiac arrest or severe hypoxia. It is characterized by slow, irregular, and minimal cardiac activity. The prognosis in patients with agonal rhythm is generally poor, but immediate and aggressive resuscitation efforts are essential for any chance of recovery. Recognizing this rhythm is crucial for healthcare providers as it signals the need for urgent life-saving interventions.

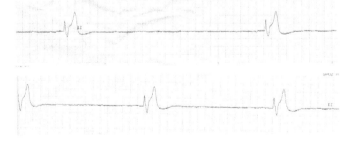

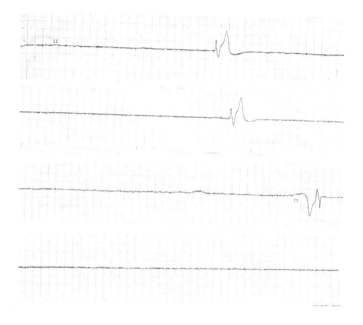

# XIV-ST SEGMENT ABNORMALITIES AND QT PROLONGATION

1. ST Elevation and Depression
2. Prolonged QT and QT Interval Correction
3. Hypercalcemia and Hypocalcemia

## 1-ST Elevation and Depression

The ST segment on an electrocardiogram (ECG) represents the period between ventricular depolarization and repolarization. Abnormalities in this segment can indicate various cardiac conditions, most notably ischemia or infarction.

### ST Elevation:

Description: Elevation of the ST segment above the baseline.

ECG Characteristics: The segment is typically elevated >1mm (about 0.04 in) in two contiguous leads.

Clinical Significance: Often indicative of acute myocardial infarction, particularly in the context of chest pain. It can also be seen in conditions like pericarditis or a ventricular aneurysm.

Management: ST elevation MI (STEMI) is a medical emergency requiring immediate intervention, often including reperfusion therapy.

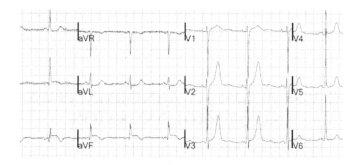

## ST Depression:

Description: Depression of the ST segment below the baseline.

ECG Characteristics: Horizontal or down sloping ST depression is considered more significant than upsloping.

Clinical Significance: Can indicate myocardial ischemia, especially if occurring during chest pain or exertion. Also seen in conditions like digitalis toxicity or hypokalemia.

Management: Depends on the underlying cause; in the case of ischemia, management includes anti-ischemic therapy and cardiac evaluation.

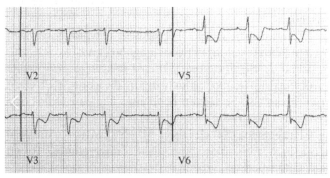

# 2-QT Prolongation and QT Interval Correction

Description: The QT interval on an ECG represents the total time for ventricular depolarization and repolarization.

Prolongation of the QT interval is a risk factor for serious arrhythmias.

ECG Characteristics: Measured from the beginning of the QRS complex to the end of the T wave. A prolonged QT is generally considered to be >440ms in men and >460ms in women.

### Causes:

Congenital: Long QT Syndrome, a genetic condition.

Acquired: Medications (especially certain antiarrhythmics, antidepressants, antipsychotics), electrolyte imbalances (like hypokalemia, hypomagnesemia), and other medical conditions.

Clinical Implications: Prolonged QT can lead to Torsade de Pointes, a type of polymorphic ventricular tachycardia, which can degenerate into ventricular fibrillation.

### QT Interval Correction

Definition

The QT interval on an electrocardiogram (ECG) represents the total time taken for ventricular depolarization and repolarization. Because the QT interval varies with heart rate, it is often corrected for heart rate to provide a more standardized measure, known as the corrected QT interval (QTc).

### Importance of QT Correction

Rate Dependence: The QT interval lengthens at slower heart rates and shortens at faster rates. Correction is necessary to determine if the QT interval is genuinely prolonged.

Risk Assessment: An abnormally long QTc interval can indicate an increased risk of certain types of ventricular tachyarrhythmias, including Torsade de Pointes.

### Methods of QT Correction
### Bazett's Formula:

Formula: $QTc = QT / \sqrt{RR}$

RR Interval: Measured in seconds, it is the interval between two consecutive R waves.

Usage: Widely used but can be less accurate at very high or low heart rates.

**Other Formulas:**

**Fridericia's Formula:** $QTc = QT / (RR^{(1/3)})$

**Framingham Formula**: $QTc = QT + 0.154 * (1 - RR)$

These formulas may offer more accuracy over a wider range of heart rates.

Practical Example of Calculation

Example: Suppose an ECG shows a QT interval of 400 milliseconds, and the heart rate is 60 beats per minute.

Calculating RR Interval: Heart rate of 60 bpm corresponds to an RR interval of 1 second (since 60 seconds divided by 60 beats = 1 second).

Using Bazett's Formula:

$QTc = 400$ ms $/ \sqrt{1 \text{ second}}$

$QTc = 400$ ms $/ 1$

$QTc = 400$ ms

Interpretation: A QTc of 400 ms is generally considered within the normal range. The normal QTc is usually less than 440 ms in men and less than 460 ms in women.

**Considerations**

Clinical Context: It's essential to interpret the QTc in the context of the patient's overall clinical picture, including medications, electrolyte levels, and medical history.

Limitations of Formulas: Each correction formula has its limitations, and discrepancies can arise, especially at extreme heart rates.

**Summary**

Correcting the QT interval for heart rate is a crucial step in accurately assessing the risk of arrhythmias associated with QT prolongation. Bazett's formula is commonly used, but it's essential to be aware of its limitations and consider using alternative formulas or clinical judgment in certain situations.

## 3-Hypercalcemia and Hypocalcemia

Hypercalcemia and hypocalcemia are conditions characterized by abnormal calcium levels in the blood. Calcium plays a critical role in various bodily functions, including bone health, muscle contractions, and nerve signaling.

### Hypercalcemia

Definition: Hypercalcemia is a condition where the calcium level in the blood is higher than normal. The normal range is typically 8.5 to 10.2 mg (about the weight of a grain of table salt)/dL (2.12 to 2.55 mmol/L).

Causes:

Hyperparathyroidism: The most common cause, where the parathyroid glands secrete too much parathyroid hormone, increasing calcium levels.

Cancer: Certain types of cancer can increase calcium levels either by metastasis to bones or by secretion of calcium-regulating hormones.

Other Causes: Include prolonged immobilization, excessive calcium or vitamin D intake, certain medications, and other endocrine disorders.

Symptoms: Fatigue, muscle weakness, increased thirst and urination, nausea and vomiting, constipation, confusion, and in severe cases, cardiac arrhythmias.

**ECG Changes: Shortened QT interval, widened T waves.**

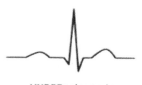

**HYPERcalcaemia**

Treatment:

Immediate: IV fluids, bisphosphonates, and corticosteroids, depending on the severity and underlying cause.

Long-Term: Addressing the underlying cause, dietary modifications, and medication management.

**Hypocalcemia**

Definition: Hypocalcemia is characterized by abnormally low levels of calcium in the blood.

Causes:

Hypoparathyroidism: Reduced production of parathyroid hormone, leading to decreased calcium levels.

Vitamin D Deficiency: Limits calcium absorption.

Renal Disease: Impairs calcium regulation.

Other Causes: Include magnesium deficiency, pancreatitis, and certain medications.

Symptoms: Muscle cramps and spasms (tetany), numbness and tingling in the fingers, convulsions, fatigue, and, in severe cases, cardiac arrhythmias.

**ECG Changes: Prolonged QT interval, prolonged ST segment.**

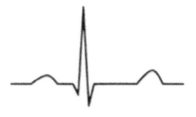

**HYPOcalcaemia**

Treatment:
Immediate: IV calcium for acute cases, especially if symptomatic.
Long-Term: Oral calcium and vitamin D supplements, dietary changes, and addressing underlying causes.

Summary
Both hypercalcemia and hypocalcemia are significant electrolyte disturbances with potentially serious consequences. They can impact various body systems, notably the cardiovascular and nervous systems, and require prompt and appropriate management. Their treatment and management depend heavily on the underlying cause and the severity of the condition. Monitoring and addressing calcium levels are crucial parts of managing various medical conditions, particularly those involving the parathyroid glands and kidneys.

# XV-Artifacts and Disturbances in EKG Interpretation

1.  Artifacts
2.  Electrical Disturbances and Device Interference

Introduction

Artifacts and disturbances in electrocardiogram (EKG) interpretation are non-cardiac factors that can affect the EKG tracing. These extraneous signals can mimic or obscure cardiac pathology, leading to misinterpretation. Understanding and identifying these artifacts is crucial for accurate EKG analysis.

## 1- Artifacts

Definition: Movement artifacts occur when patient movement produces erratic, non-cardiac signals on the EKG.

Characteristics:

ECG Appearance: Irregular, jagged lines that do not correlate with typical ECG patterns.

Common Causes: Patient movement, shivering, tremors, or adjusting position during the EKG recording.

### Impact on Interpretation:

Misinterpretation: These artifacts can be mistaken for cardiac arrhythmias or ischemic changes.

Resolution: Ensuring the patient is calm and still, proper electrode attachment and a comfortable environment can minimize these artifacts.

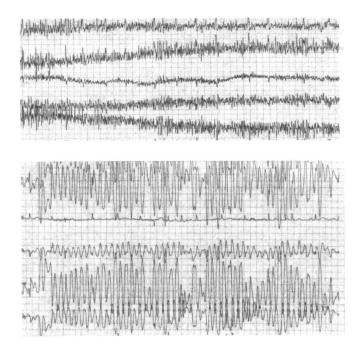

## 2-Electrical Disturbances and Device Interference

### Electrical Disturbances:

Sources: External electrical sources such as lights, electrical cables, or other medical equipment.

ECG Appearance: Regular, spiking or undulating patterns that are consistent and unrelated to cardiac rhythm.

Resolution: Removing or distancing the interference source, ensuring proper grounding of EKG equipment, and using shielded cables can help.

### Device Interference:

Types:

**Cell Phones and Electronic Devices: Can introduce erratic spikes or signals.**

Pacemakers: Present as regular, small spikes on the EKG, indicating pacing activity. This is a normal finding for patients with pacemakers but must be differentiated from other types of electrical interference.

**ECG Appearance: Depending on the device, interference can appear as regular or irregular spikes or noise.**

Impact: Can mask or mimic cardiac events, particularly arrhythmias.

Resolution: Patients should be advised to turn off or distance electronic devices during EKG recording.

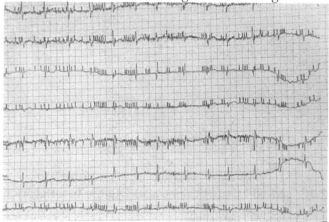

Summary

Recognizing artifacts and disturbances is a critical skill in EKG interpretation. These non-cardiac sources of interference can lead to misdiagnosis if not identified and accounted for. By understanding the common sources and appearances of these artifacts, clinicians can more accurately interpret EKG findings and make informed decisions about patient care. In cases of doubt, repeating the EKG under controlled conditions or using additional diagnostic tools may be necessary to clarify the patient's cardiac status.

# Practical Applications

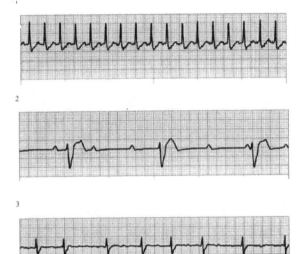

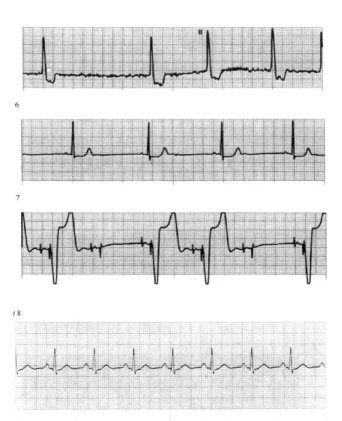

6

7

⊦ 8

9

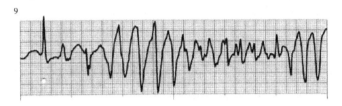

10

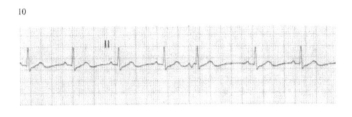

4

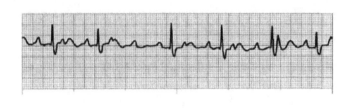

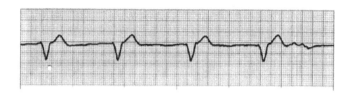

# 2

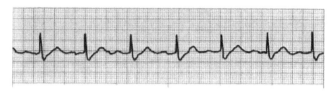

# 3

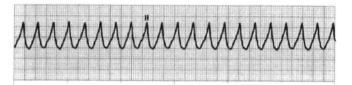

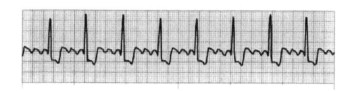

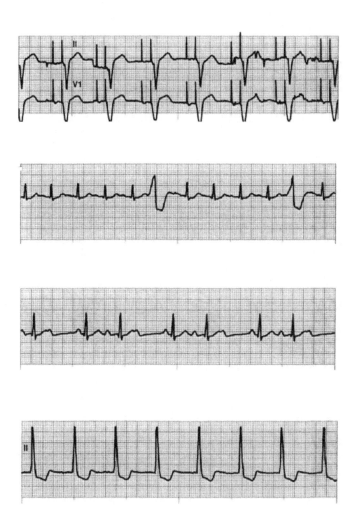

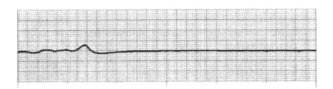

10

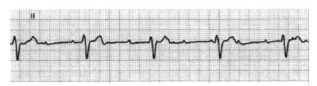

11

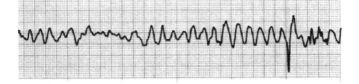

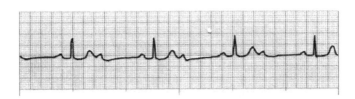

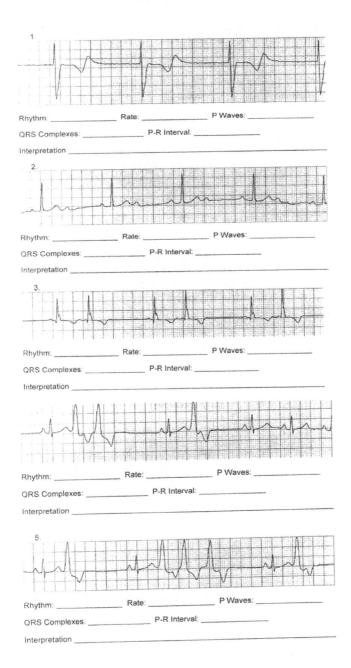

**1.**

Rhythm: _____ Rate: _____ P Waves: _____

QRS Complexes: _____ P-R Interval: _____

Interpretation _____

**2.**

Rhythm: _____ Rate: _____ P Waves: _____

QRS Complexes: _____ P-R Interval: _____

Interpretation _____

**3.**

Rhythm: _____ Rate: _____ P Waves: _____

QRS Complexes: _____ P-R Interval: _____

Interpretation _____

Rhythm: _____ Rate: _____ P Waves: _____

QRS Complexes: _____ P-R Interval: _____

Interpretation _____

**5.**

Rhythm: _____ Rate: _____ P Waves: _____

QRS Complexes: _____ P-R Interval: _____

Interpretation _____

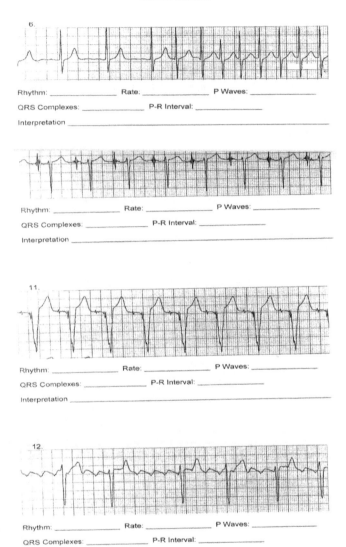

6.

Rhythm: _____ Rate: _____ P Waves: _____

QRS Complexes: _____ P-R Interval: _____

Interpretation _____

Rhythm: _____ Rate: _____ P Waves: _____

QRS Complexes: _____ P-R Interval: _____

Interpretation _____

11.

Rhythm: _____ Rate: _____ P Waves: _____

QRS Complexes: _____ P-R Interval: _____

Interpretation _____

12.

Rhythm: _____ Rate: _____ P Waves: _____

QRS Complexes: _____ P-R Interval: _____

Interpretation _____

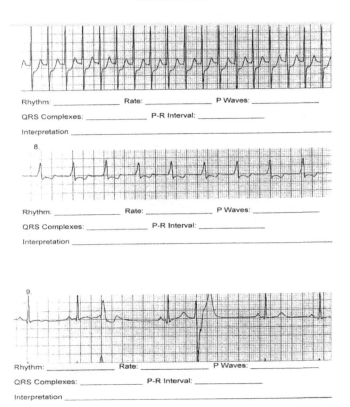

Rhythm: _____ Rate: _____ P Waves: _____

QRS Complexes: _____ P-R Interval: _____

Interpretation _____

8.

Rhythm: _____ Rate: _____ P Waves: _____

QRS Complexes: _____ P-R Interval: _____

Interpretation _____

9.

Rhythm: _____ Rate: _____ P Waves: _____

QRS Complexes: _____ P-R Interval: _____

Interpretation _____

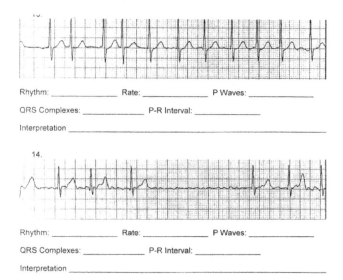

Rhythm: _____ Rate: _____ P Waves: _____

QRS Complexes: _____ P-R Interval: _____

Interpretation _____

Rhythm: _____ Rate: _____ P Waves: _____

QRS Complexes: _____ P-R Interval: _____

Interpretation _____

All strips are six (6) seconds in length.

1.

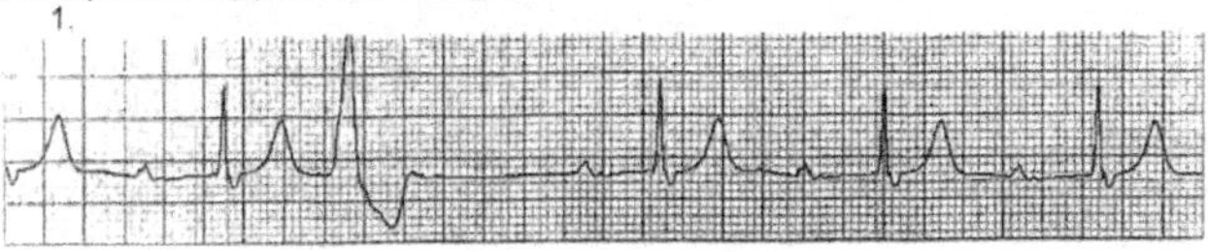

Rhythm: _____ Rate: _____ P Waves: _____

QRS Complexes: _____ P-R Interval: _____

Interpretation _____

2.

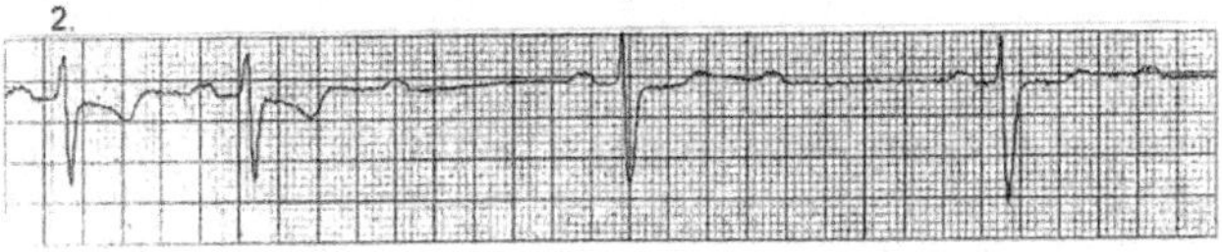

Rhythm: _____ Rate: _____ P Waves: _____

QRS Complexes: _____ P-R Interval: _____

Interpretation _____

3.

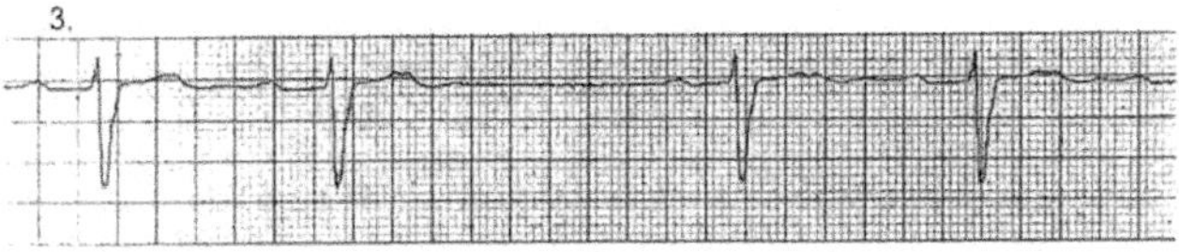

Rhythm: _____ Rate: _____ P Waves: _____

QRS Complexes: _____ P-R Interval: _____

Interpretation

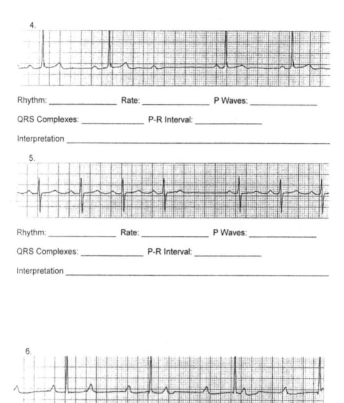

4.

Rhythm: _____ Rate: _____ P Waves: _____

QRS Complexes: _____ P-R Interval: _____

Interpretation _____

5.

Rhythm: _____ Rate: _____ P Waves: _____

QRS Complexes: _____ P-R Interval: _____

Interpretation _____

6.

Rhythm: _____ Rate: _____ P Waves: _____

QRS Complexes: _____ P-R Interval: _____

Interpretation _____

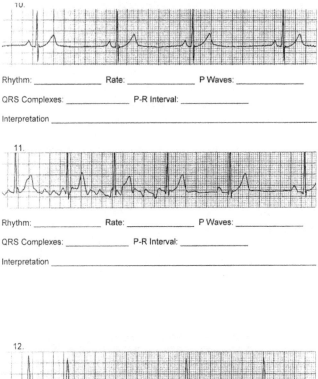

10.

Rhythm: _____ Rate: _____ P Waves: _____

QRS Complexes: _____ P-R Interval: _____

Interpretation _____

11.

Rhythm: _____ Rate: _____ P Waves: _____

QRS Complexes: _____ P-R Interval: _____

Interpretation _____

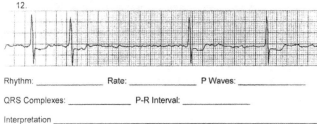

12.

Rhythm: _____ Rate: _____ P Waves: _____

QRS Complexes: _____ P-R Interval: _____

Interpretation _____

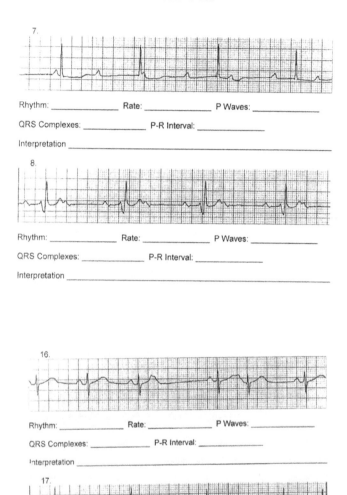

7.

Rhythm: _____ Rate: _____ P Waves: _____

QRS Complexes: _____ P-R Interval: _____

Interpretation _____

8.

Rhythm: _____ Rate: _____ P Waves: _____

QRS Complexes: _____ P-R Interval: _____

Interpretation _____

16.

Rhythm: _____ Rate: _____ P Waves: _____

QRS Complexes: _____ P-R Interval: _____

Interpretation _____

17.

Rhythm: _____ Rate: _____ P Waves: _____

QRS Complexes: _____ P-R Interval: _____

Interpretation _____

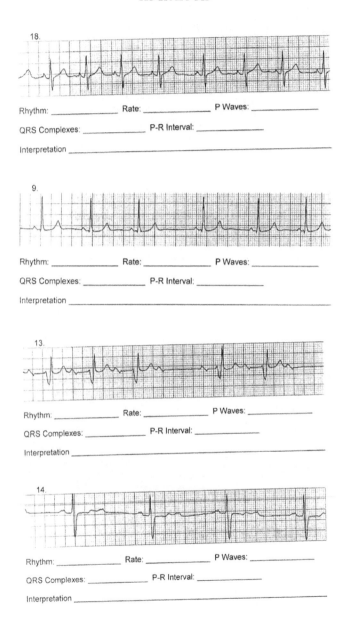

18.

Rhythm: _____ Rate: _____ P Waves: _____

QRS Complexes: _____ P-R Interval: _____

Interpretation _____

9.

Rhythm: _____ Rate: _____ P Waves: _____

QRS Complexes: _____ P-R Interval: _____

Interpretation _____

13.

Rhythm: _____ Rate: _____ P Waves: _____

QRS Complexes: _____ P-R Interval: _____

Interpretation _____

14.

Rhythm: _____ Rate: _____ P Waves: _____

QRS Complexes: _____ P-R Interval: _____

Interpretation _____

# ROCK LOUIS

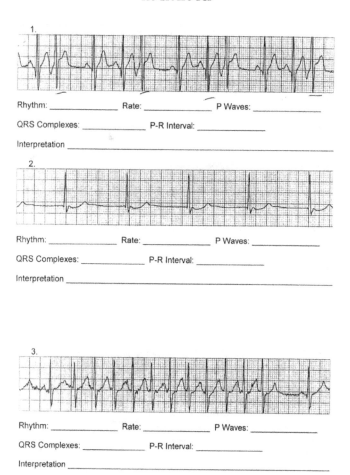

**1.**

Rhythm: _____ Rate: _____ P Waves: _____

QRS Complexes: _____ P-R Interval: _____

Interpretation _____

**2.**

Rhythm: _____ Rate: _____ P Waves: _____

QRS Complexes: _____ P-R Interval: _____

Interpretation _____

**3.**

Rhythm: _____ Rate: _____ P Waves: _____

QRS Complexes: _____ P-R Interval: _____

Interpretation _____

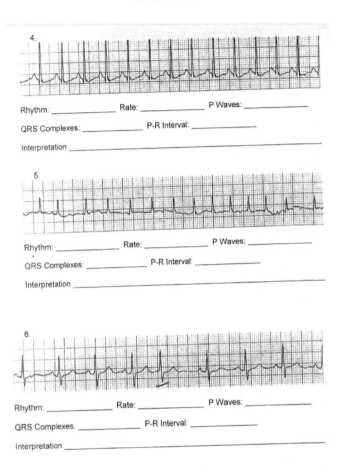

4.

Rhythm: _____ Rate: _____ P Waves: _____

QRS Complexes: _____ P-R Interval: _____

Interpretation _____

5.

Rhythm: _____ Rate: _____ P Waves: _____

QRS Complexes: _____ P-R Interval: _____

Interpretation _____

6.

Rhythm: _____ Rate: _____ P Waves: _____

QRS Complexes: _____ P-R Interval: _____

Interpretation _____

10.

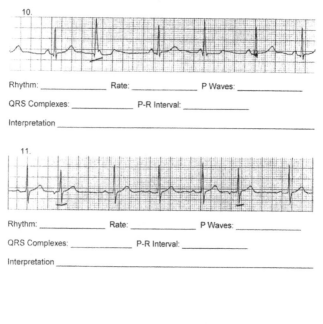

Rhythm: _____ Rate: _____ P Waves: _____

QRS Complexes: _____ P-R Interval: _____

Interpretation _____

11.

Rhythm: _____ Rate: _____ P Waves: _____

QRS Complexes: _____ P-R Interval: _____

Interpretation _____

12.

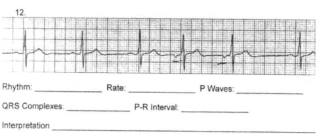

Rhythm: _____ Rate: _____ P Waves: _____

QRS Complexes: _____ P-R Interval: _____

Interpretation _____

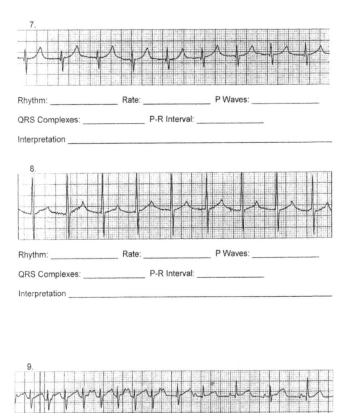

**7.**

Rhythm: _____ Rate: _____ P Waves: _____

QRS Complexes: _____ P-R Interval: _____

Interpretation _____

**8.**

Rhythm: _____ Rate: _____ P Waves: _____

QRS Complexes: _____ P-R Interval: _____

Interpretation _____

**9.**

Rhythm: _____ Rate: _____ P Waves: _____

QRS Complexes: _____ P-R Interval: _____

Interpretation _____

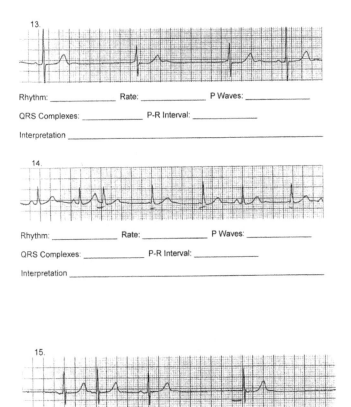

13.

Rhythm: _____ Rate: _____ P Waves: _____

QRS Complexes: _____ P-R Interval: _____

Interpretation _____

14.

Rhythm: _____ Rate: _____ P Waves: _____

QRS Complexes: _____ P-R Interval: _____

Interpretation _____

15.

Rhythm: _____ Rate: _____ P Waves: _____

QRS Complexes: _____ P-R Interval: _____

Interpretation _____

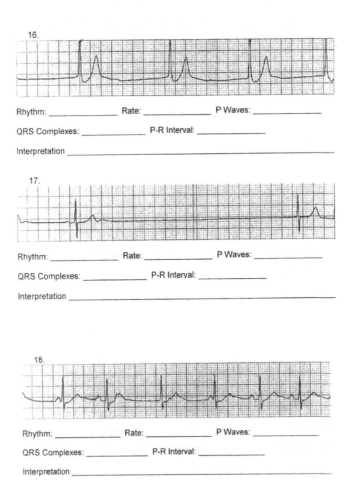

16.

Rhythm: _____ Rate: _____ P Waves: _____

QRS Complexes: _____ P-R Interval: _____

Interpretation _____

17.

Rhythm: _____ Rate: _____ P Waves: _____

QRS Complexes: _____ P-R Interval: _____

Interpretation _____

18.

Rhythm: _____ Rate: _____ P Waves: _____

QRS Complexes: _____ P-R Interval: _____

Interpretation _____

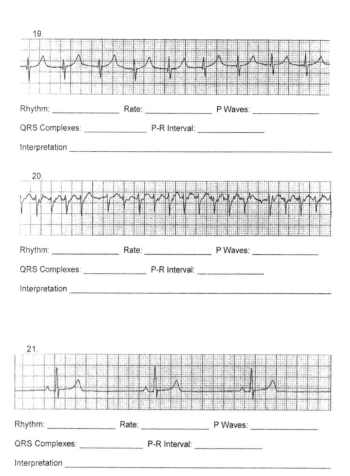

19.

Rhythm: _____ Rate: _____ P Waves: _____

QRS Complexes: _____ P-R Interval: _____

Interpretation _____

20.

Rhythm: _____ Rate: _____ P Waves: _____

QRS Complexes: _____ P-R Interval: _____

Interpretation _____

21.

Rhythm: _____ Rate: _____ P Waves: _____

QRS Complexes: _____ P-R Interval: _____

Interpretation _____

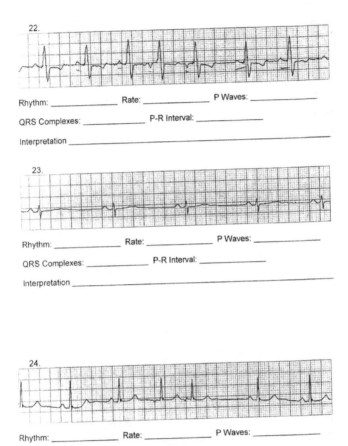

22.

Rhythm: _____ Rate: _____ P Waves: _____

QRS Complexes: _____ P-R Interval: _____

Interpretation _____

23.

Rhythm: _____ Rate: _____ P Waves: _____

QRS Complexes: _____ P-R Interval: _____

Interpretation _____

24.

Rhythm: _____ Rate: _____ P Waves: _____

QRS Complexes: _____ P-R Interval: _____

Interpretation _____

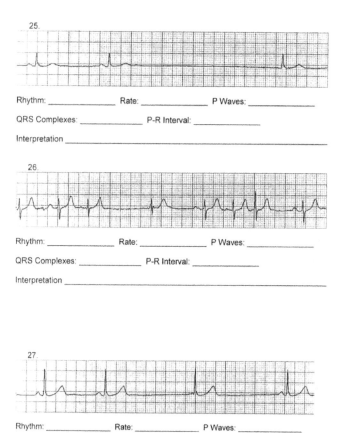

25.

Rhythm: _____ Rate: _____ P Waves: _____

QRS Complexes: _____ P-R Interval: _____

Interpretation _____

26.

Rhythm: _____ Rate: _____ P Waves: _____

QRS Complexes: _____ P-R Interval: _____

Interpretation _____

27.

Rhythm: _____ Rate: _____ P Waves: _____

QRS Complexes: _____ P-R Interval: _____

Interpretation _____

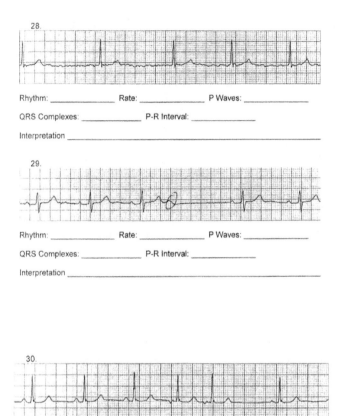

**28.**

Rhythm: _____ Rate: _____ P Waves: _____

QRS Complexes: _____ P-R Interval: _____

Interpretation _____

**29.**

Rhythm: _____ Rate: _____ P Waves: _____

QRS Complexes: _____ P-R Interval: _____

Interpretation _____

**30.**

Rhythm: _____ Rate: _____ P Waves: _____

QRS Complexes: _____ P-R Interval: _____

Interpretation _____

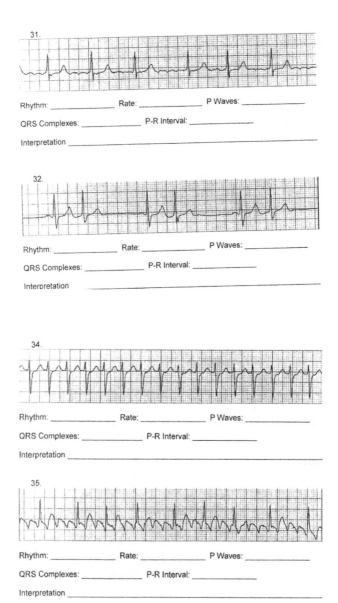

31.

Rhythm: _____ Rate: _____ P Waves: _____

QRS Complexes: _____ P-R Interval: _____

Interpretation _____

32.

Rhythm: _____ Rate: _____ P Waves: _____

QRS Complexes: _____ P-R Interval: _____

Interpretation _____

34.

Rhythm: _____ Rate: _____ P Waves: _____

QRS Complexes: _____ P-R Interval: _____

Interpretation _____

35.

Rhythm: _____ Rate: _____ P Waves: _____

QRS Complexes: _____ P-R Interval: _____

Interpretation _____

36.

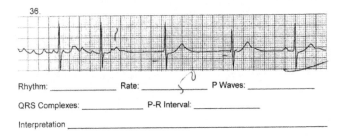

Rhythm: _____ Rate: _____ P Waves: _____

QRS Complexes: _____ P-R Interval: _____

Interpretation _____

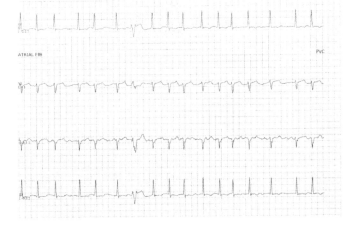

ATRIAL FIB

PVC

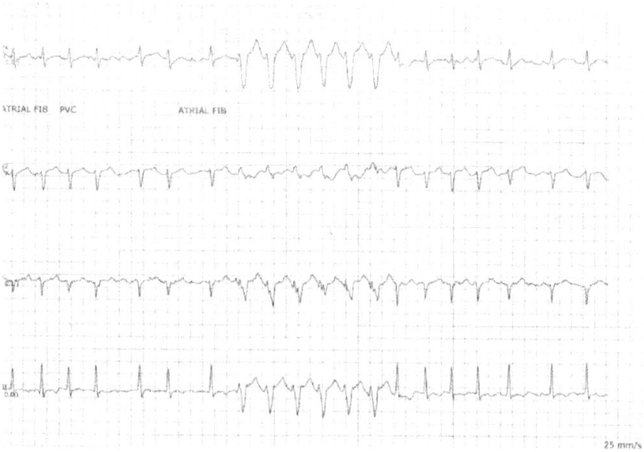
ATRIAL FIB PVC
ATRIAL FIB
25 mm/s

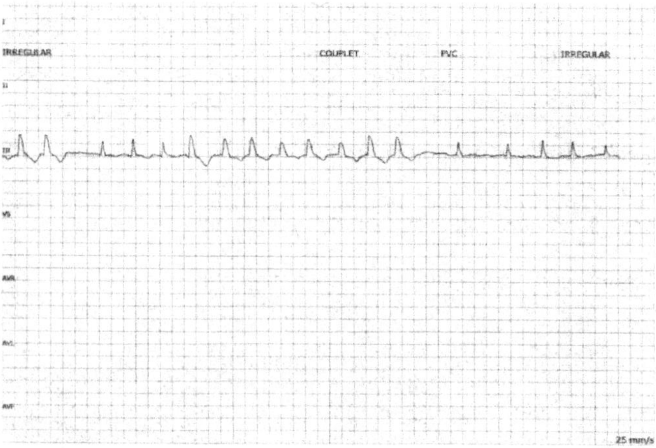
IRREGULAR
COUPLET
PVC
IRREGULAR
25 mm/s

# ROCK LOUIS

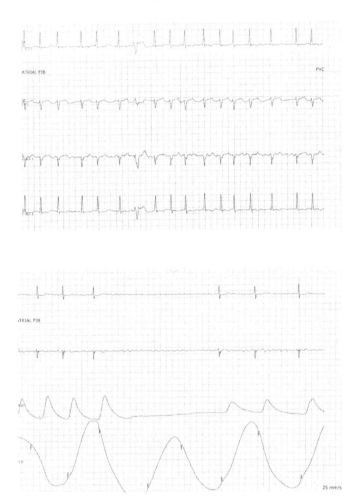

155

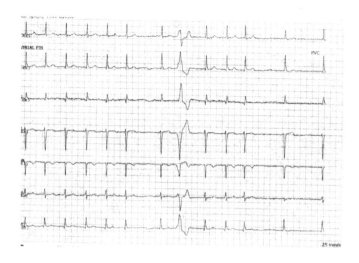

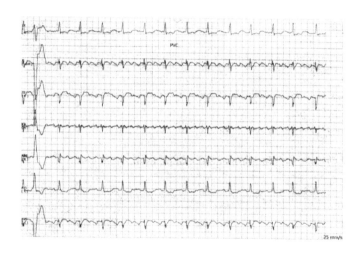

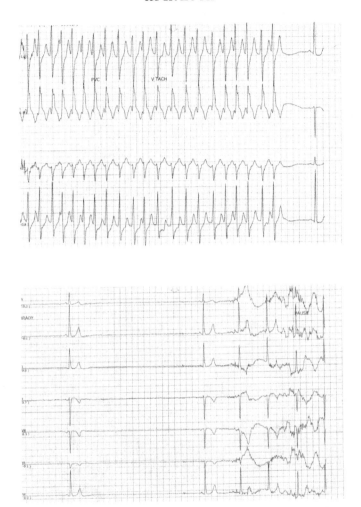

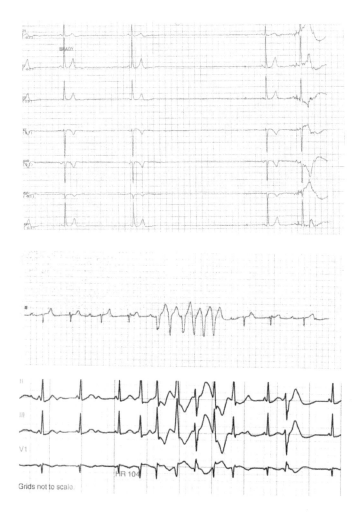

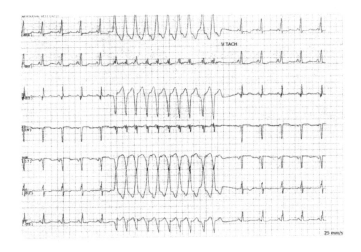

V. TACH

25 mm/s

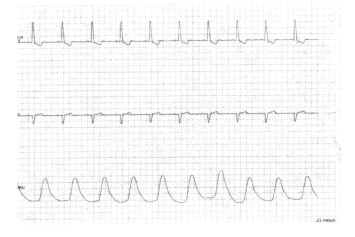

25 mm/s

159

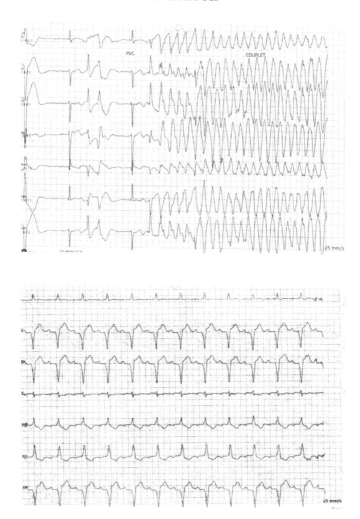

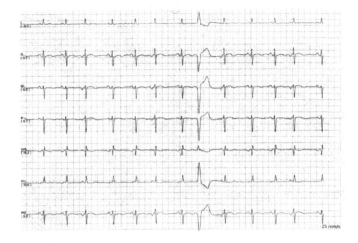

Made in the USA
Middletown, DE
24 August 2024